HANDBOOK OF DERMATOLOGY

HANDBOOK OF DERMATOLOGY

Second Edition

G Ilangovan MD DD DIH PhD
Emeritus Professor of Dermatology
The Tamil Nadu Dr MGR Medical University
Former Director of Medical Education
Senior Consultant Dermatologist
Government of Tamil Nadu
India

JAYPEE

JAYPEE BROTHERS MEDICAL PUBLISHERS (P) LTD

New Delhi • London • Philadelphia • Panama

Jaypee Brothers Medical Publishers (P) Ltd

Jaypee Brothers Medical Publishers (P) Ltd.
4838/24, Ansari Road, Daryaganj
New Delhi 110 002, India
Phone: +91-11-43574357
Fax: +91-11-43574314
jaypee@jaypeebrothers.com
www.jaypeebrothers.com
www.jaypeedigital.com

J.P. Medical Ltd.,
83 Victoria Street London
SW1H 0HW UK
Phone: +44 (0) 20 3170 8910
Fax: +44 (0) 20 3008 6180
info@jpmedpub.com
www.jpmedpub.com

Jaypee-Highlights Medical Publishers Inc.
City of Knowledge, Bld. 237, Clayton
Panama City, Panama
Phone: +50-73-010496
Fax: +50-73-010499
cservice@jphmedical.com
www.jphmedical.com

Handbook of Dermatology

First Edition: 1995

Second Edition: **2013**

ISBN: 978-93-5090-454-1

Printed at Samrat Offset Pvt. Ltd.

PREFACE

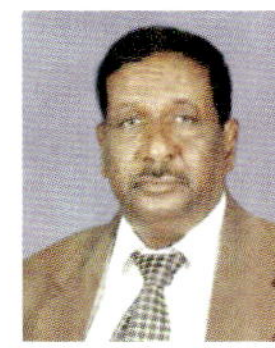

This introduction to dermatology has been written as a reference tool for undergraduate students, postgraduate residents, fellows, and will also be useful for practitioners and nurses.

G Ilangovan

ACKNOWLEDGMENT

I am greatly indebted to my family members and my friends, who encouraged me to write this book.

CONTENTS

1. ACANTHOSIS NIGRICANS

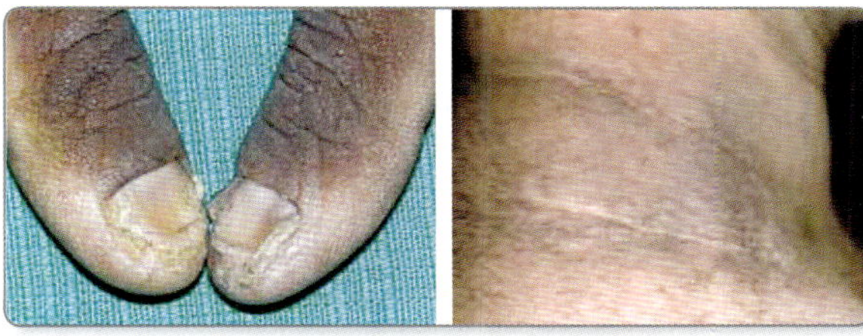

Acanthosis nigricans

Acanthosis nigricans, a cutaneous maker of internal malignancy characterized by thickening, pigmentation and papillomatosis of the skin particularly over body folds and mucous membranes.

It typically occurs in individuals younger than age 40, may be genetically inherited, and is associated with obesity or endocrinopathies such as hypothyroidism or hyperthyroidism, acromegaly, polycystic ovary disease, insulin-resistant diabetes, or Cushing's disease.

TYPES

1. Hereditary benign acanthosis nigricans.
2. Benign acanthosis nigricans. For example: Addisons disease, Cushing's disease.
3. Pseudoacanthosis nigricans in obesity.
4. Drug-induced acanthosis nigricans: Nicotinic acid, oral contraceptives, corticosteroids.
5. Malignant acanthosis nigricans: Adenocarcioma.

Treatment: 1. Treatment towards the underlying cause
2. Topical tretinoin 0.1%

2. ACNE VULGARIS

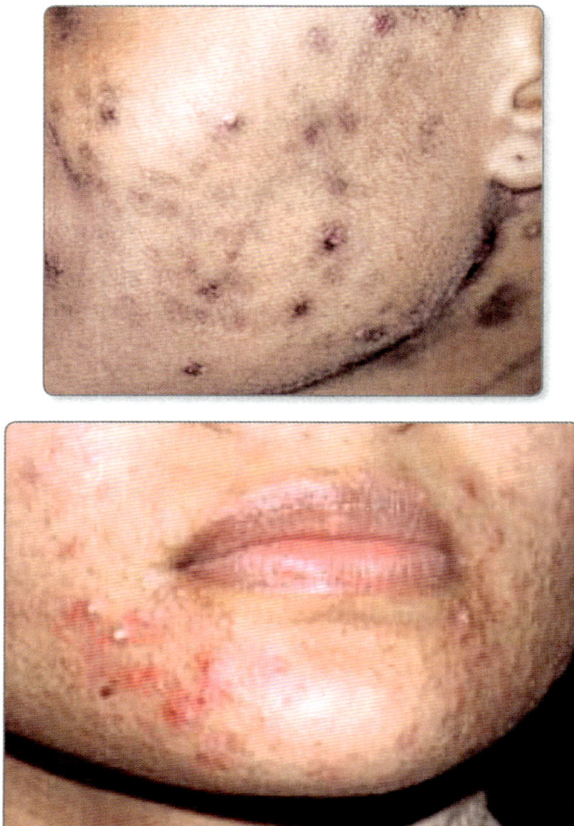

Acne vulgaris

A disease of teenage but even adults can be affected. Both sexes are affected equally. It is a chronic inflammatory disease of pilosebaceous unit. The clinical picture varies from comedones, papules, pustules, cysts, nodules and even scars over face, neck, upper trunk. It occurs primarly over seborrheic areas of skin.

Comedo (Black head) is the basic lesion of acne.

Clinical varieties: Acne vulgaris, atrophic acne, steroid acne, cystic acne, acne conglobata.

ETIOPATHOGENESIS

Hereditary Factor

Androgenic stimulation of sebaceous glands.

Colonization of follicle by *Propionibacterium acnes* which metabolizes sebum to produce fatty acids which are chemotactic to the components of inflammation.

Emotional factors play a role.

Treatment Systemic: Tetracycline, minocycline, clindamycin, erythomycin, sulfonamide.

Topical: Benozoyl peroxide, retinoic acid, sulfur, clindamycin, erythromycin.

Laser acne therapy.

3. ADENOMA SEBACEUM

(BOURNEVILLE'S DISEASE)

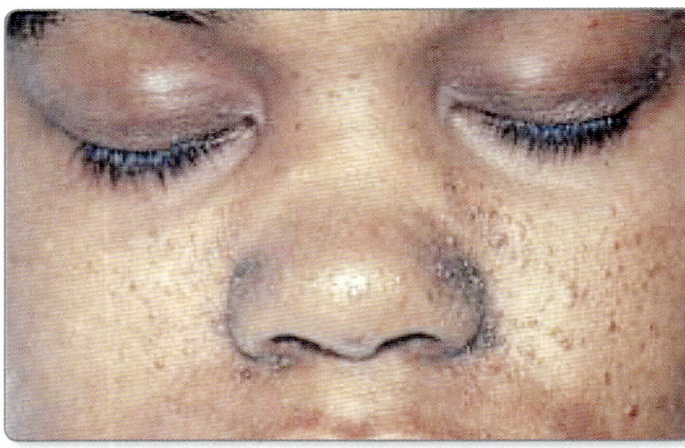

Adenoma sebaceum

Tuberous sclerosis is a group of two genetic disorders that affect the skin, brain/nervous system, kidneys, and heart, and cause tumors to grow. The diseases are named after a tuber- or root-shaped growth in the brain. It is one of the neurocutaneous syndromes.

AUTOSOMAL DOMINANT

Tuberous Sclerosis (Epiloia)

Epi–epliepsy, loi–low intelligence; a–adenoma sebaceum. Adenoma sebaceum is a pinhead size, discrete, waxy papules over face. Other manifestations are: Shagreen patch, oral papillomatosis, ash-leaf macule, skin fibromas, cafe au lait spots.

Cerebral classification - potato-like nodules, retinal tumors (phakomas) renal hamartomas, bone cysts are seen.

Investigations:

X-ray skull, CAT scan, X-ray hands and feet, Wood's lamp examination, fundoscopy.

4. AIDS

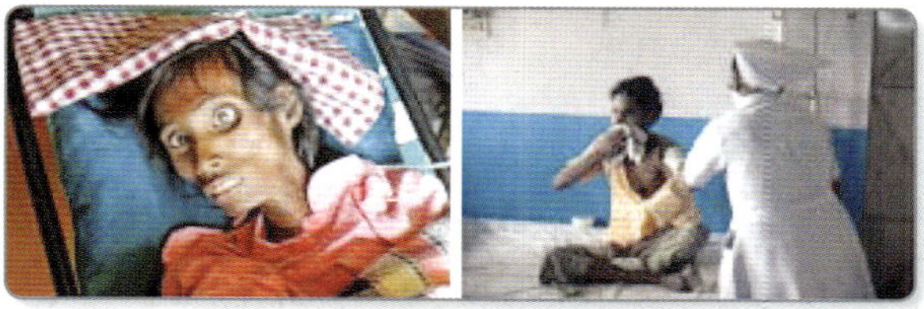

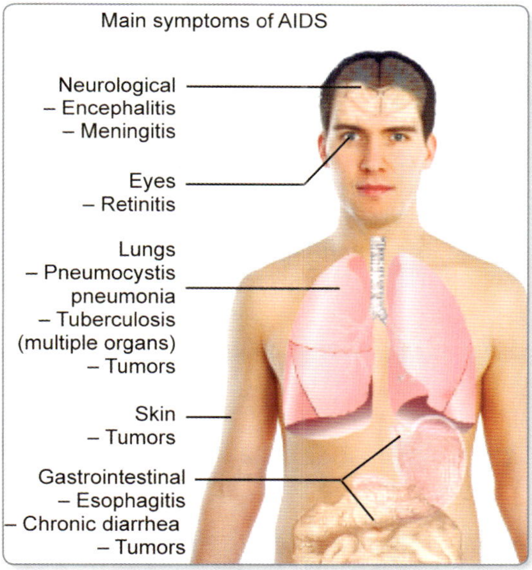

AIDS

Acquired immune deficiency syndrome or acquired immunodeficiency syndrome (AIDS) is a disease of the human immune system caused by the Human immunodeficiency virus (HIV) This condition progressively reduces the effectiveness of the immune system and leaves individuals susceptible to opportunistic infections and tumors. HIV is transmitted through direct contact of a mucous membrane or the bloodstream with a bodily fluid containing HIV such as blood, semen, vaginal fluid, preseminal fluid, and breast milk. This transmission is due to anal, vaginal or oral sex, blood transfusion, contaminated hypodermic needles, exchange between mother and baby during pregnancy, childbirth, breastfeeding or other exposure to one of the above bodily fluids.

The symptoms of AIDS are primarily the result of conditions that do not normally develop in individuals with healthy immune systems. Most of these conditions are infections caused by bacteria, viruses, fungi and parasites that are normally controlled by the elements of the immune system that HIV damages.

1. **Cardinal findings:**
   - Kaposi sarcoma
   - *Pneumocystis carinii* pneumonia.
   - Toxoplasma encephalitis
   - Esophageal candidiasis
   - Cytomegalovirus retinitis
2. **Associated findings:**

   Weight loss (recent, unexplained) of more than 10% of baseline body weight.

   Fever (continuous or intermittent) for more than 1 month; diarrhea (continuous or intermittent) for more than 1 month; ulcers (genital or perianal) for more than 1 month; cough for more than 1 month; neurological complaints or findings generalized lymphadenopathy (extrainguinal).

   Drug reactions (previously not seen), e.g. to thiacetazone or sulfonamides.

   Skin infections (severe or recurrent), e.g. warts, dermatophytes, folliculitis.
3. **Cutaneous manifestations of AIDS:**

   Superficial fungal infections: Candidiasis, dermatophytosis.

   Disseminatied fungal and protozoal infections: *Cryptococcus neoformans* infection, histoplasmosis, amoebiasis, *Pneumocystis carinii* pneumonia, coccidiodomycosis.

   Bacterial and mycobacterial infections: *Staphylococcus aureus* infection, *Mycobacterium tuberculosis* and *M. leprae* infection, actinomycosis.

Viral: Human papillomavirus infection, molluscum contagiosum, herpes simplex virus infections, herpes zoster (multidermatomal).
Pruritic papular and follicur eruptions: Insect bite reactions, prurigo nodularis.
Papulosquamous disorders: Seborrheic dermatitis, psoriasis, Reiter's syndrome, atopic dermatitis, lichen planus.
Malignancies: Kaposi's sarcoma, squamous cell carcinoma, Basal - cell carcinoma.

4. **Epidemiological risk factors:**
   1. Present or past high-risk behavior:
      Drug injecting
      Multiple sex partners:
      Sex partner(s) with known AIDS of HIV infection.
      Sex partner(s) with known epidemiological risk factor or from an area with a high prevalence of HIV infection males having penetrative sexual intercourse with males.

The pathophysiology of AIDS is complex, as is the case with all syndromes. HIV causes AIDS by depleting $CD4^{+}$ T helper lymphocytes. This weakens the immune system and allows opportunistic infections. T lymphocytes are essential to the immune response and without them, the body cannot fight infections or kill cancerous cells. The mechanism of $CD4^{+}$ T cell depletion differs in the acute and chronic phases.

A major cause of $CD4^{+}$ T cell loss appears to result from their heightened susceptibility to apoptosis when the immune system remains activated. Although new T cells are continuously produced by the thymus to replace the ones lost, the regenerative capacity of the thymus is slowly destroyed by direct infection of its thymocytes by HIV. Eventually, the minimal number of $CD4^{+}$ T cells necessary to maintain a sufficient immune response is lost, leading to AIDS.

HIV TEST

Routinely used HIV tests for infection in neonates and infants (i.e. patients younger than 2 years) born to HIV-positive mothers, have no value because of the presence of maternal antibody to HIV in the child's blood. HIV infection can only be diagnosed by polymerase chain reaction (PCR), testing for HIV proviral DNA in the children's lymphocytes.

WHO DISEASE STAGING SYSTEM

Stage I: HIV infection is asymptomatic and not categorized as AIDS

Stage II: Includes minor mucocutaneous manifestations and recurrent upper respiratory tract infections

Stage III: Includes unexplained chronic diarrhea for longer than a month, severe bacterial infections and pulmonary tuberculosis

Stage IV: Includes toxoplasmosis of the brain, candidiasis of the esophagus, trachea, bronchi or lungs and Kaposi's sarcoma; these diseases are indicators of AIDS.

5. ALOPECIA AREATA

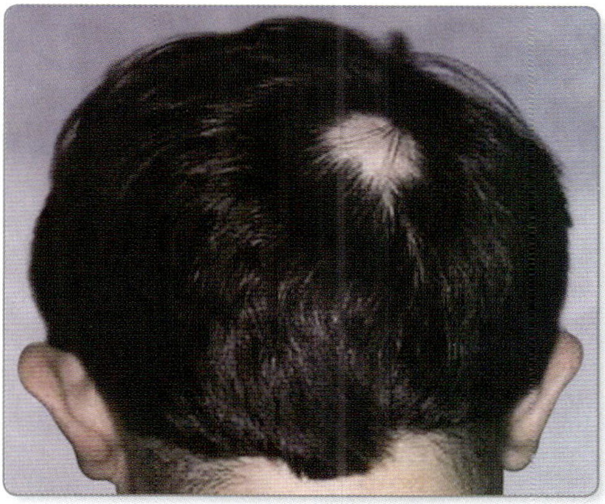

Alopecia areata

Rapid patchy loss of hair in one or several areas of scalp, beard and eyebrow.

Alopecia areata monolocularis describes baldness in only one spot. It may occur anywhere on the head.

Alopecia areata multilocularis refers to multiple areas of hair loss. If the patient loses all the hair on his scalp, the disease is then called alopecia areata totalis.

If all body hair, including pubic hair is lost, the diagnosis then becomes alopecia areata universalis.

Associated with other autoimmune disease, atopic eczema, Down's syndrome, vitiligo, thyroiditis.

Histology: Chronic lymphocytic inflammatory infiltrate around hair bulbs- "Swarm of bees" appearance.

Differential diagnosis: Trichotillomania, tinea capitis.

Treatment: Intralesional steroids, induction of contact sensitization with DNCB, PUVA therapy.

6. ANIMAL SCABIES

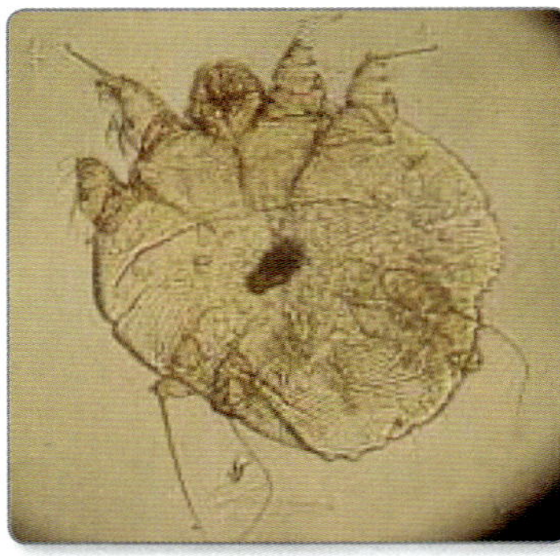

Animal scabies

Transmitted by animals which are infected by mites. Man gets infected by the pets (animals) when he comes in close contact with these animals like dogs, cats, poultry birds, horses, self-limited. No burrows. Itchy papular lesion over trunk.

AGENTS

Sarcoptes scabies var canis, Notoedres cati

Treatment: Avoid contact with animals. Treatment is like that of scabies.

7. APHTHOUS ULCER

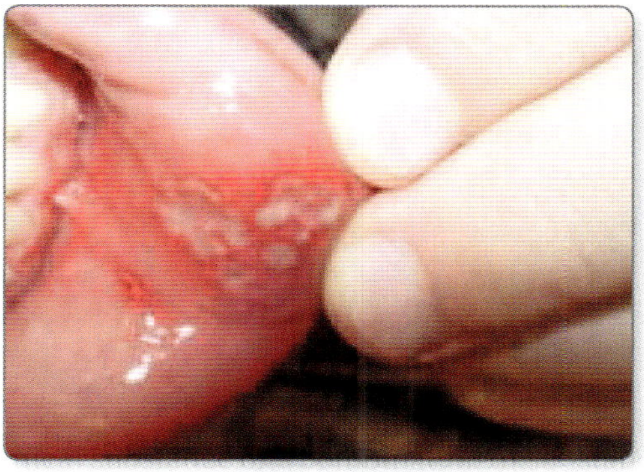

Aphthous ulcer

Mouth ulcer which presents as a painful open sore inside the mouth. Recurrent ulceration of the oral mucosa of unknown etiology. Predisposing factors: Emotional stress, vitamin B_{12} deficiency, folic acid, iron deficiency, physical trauma, dental braces, thermal injury.

Ulcers are seen over lips, tongue, buccal mucosa.

Differential diagnosis: Recurrent herpes simplex, Behcet's syndrome, bullous dermatoses like pemphigus.

Minor ulceration: 3–10 mm

Major ulcerations: Greater than 10 mm

Herpetiform ulcerations: Severe form small, numerous, 1–3 mm lesions that form clusters.

Treatment: Nonspecific. A number of different treatments exist for aphthous ulcers including: analgesics, anesthetics agents, antiseptics, anti-inflammatory agents, steroids, sucralfate, tetracycline suspension, and silver nitrate. Amlexanox paste has been found to speed healing and alleviate pain. Corticosteroid preparations containing hydrocortisone can be tried.

8. ATOPIC DERMATITIS

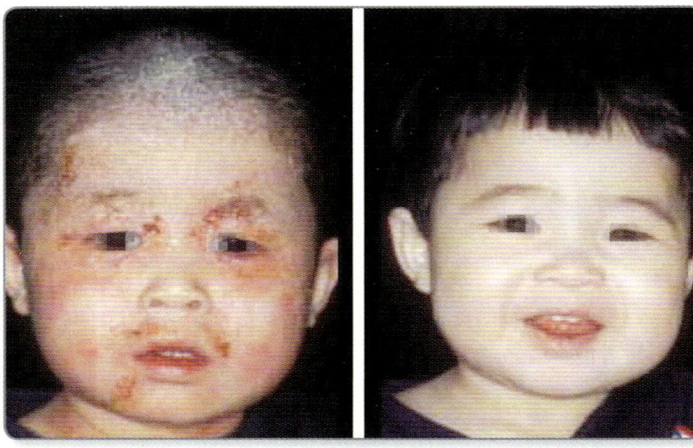

Atopic dermatitis

DEFINITION

Atopy means 'out of place' or strange. Hereditary tendency to develop allergy to food and inhalant substances manifested as eczema, asthma and hay fever (EAH syndrome), endogenous eczema.

Three stages: Infantile phase - 2 months to 2 years.
Childhood phase - 2 to 10 years.
Adolescent and adult phase - above 10 years.

Infantile type: Itchy, erythematous patches vesicles, rupture, moist crust over scalp (cardle cap), neck, forehead, wrist, extremities, diaper areas, buttocks, cubital, popliteal fossae.

Moist Type and Dry Type

Childhood types: Pruritus, scratching, exudative papular lichenification and secondary infection present. Antecubital popliteal space affected. Food allergy and feather sensitivity present.

Adult type: Erythema, scaly, papular or vesicular, lichenified plaques, present antecubital popliteal fossae, side of the neck, forehead, hands and wrist are affected.

Associated features: Dennie-Morgan fold, keratosis pilaris, Hertogue sign (thinning of lateral eyebrows). Headlight sign. White dermographism, contract infection with Staphylococcus, Kaposi's varicelliform eruption.

Treatment

Topical: Corticosteroid creams

Systemic therapy: Antihistamine, oral corticosteroids, antibiotics.

Atopic dermatitis (AD: a type of eczema) is an inflammatory, chronically relapsing, non-contagious and pruritic skin disorder.

9. BOCKHART'S IMPETIGO

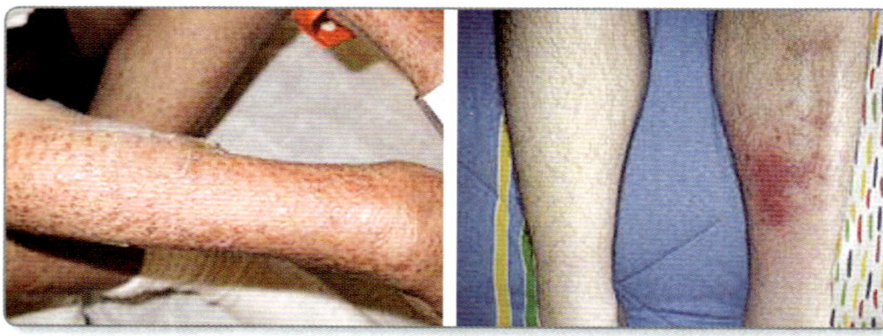

Bockhart's impetigo

Superficial contagious bacterial infection of the hair follicle caused by Staphylococcus. Pustules develop over scalp, hair margin and extremities. Superficial folliculitis with thin-walled pustules at the folliclular openings.

Treatment: Topical and systemic antibiotics.

10. CALLOSITY

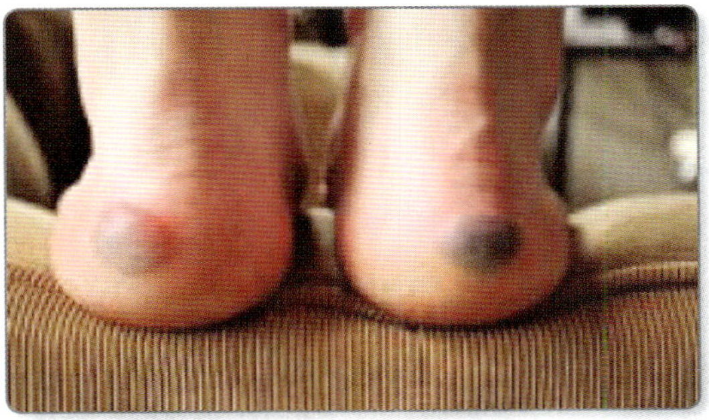

Callosity

It is a circumscribed hyperkeratosis of the skin produced by repeated or constant friction or pressure at a particular site. The center part of a callosity is the thickest, tapering to the periphery and merging with the normal skin.

Site: Palms and soles and at bony prominences such as the elbows, knees and malleoli.

Treatment: Topical keratolytics.

11. CHANCROID

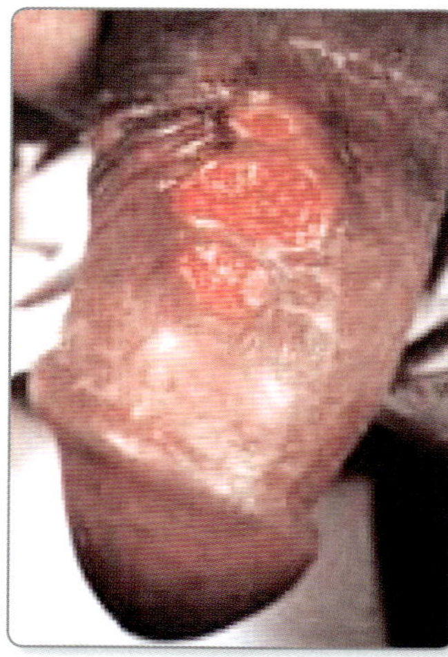

Chancroid

STD bacterial infection caused by *Haemophilus ducreyi*. Sores on the mouth, throat, lips, anus, tongue, vagina, or penis. Chancroid is a risk factor for contracting the HIV virus. The ulcer may look like a chancre, the typical sore of primary syphilis. About half of the people who are infected with a chancroid will develop enlarged inguinal lymph nodes. Painful open sores on the genitals, and in some cases, swollen and tender lymph nodes in the groin.

Treatment: Antibiotics are usually effective—Azithromycin 1.0 g (250 mg × 4 tablets) or Ciproflox 500 mg twice a day.

12. CHEILITIS

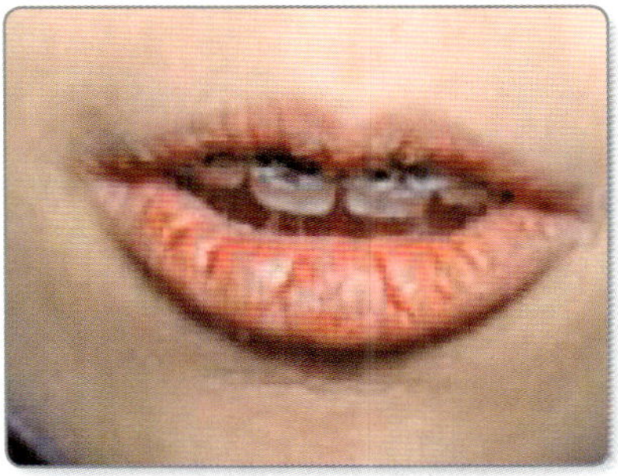

Cheilitis

Inflammatory disorder of the lips from different causes manifested by dryness, scaling, fissuring. Types:

1. Contact cheilitis: Lipstick the commonest substance incriminated, others are nailpolish, topical medicaments, sunscreens, cosmetics, mouthwashes, toothpaste, dental preparations.

   Treatment: Avoid offending agents. Mild steroids topically.
2. Actinic cheilitis: Prolonged and excessive exposure to sunlight.

   Treatment: Avoid sunlight. Topical sunscreening agents and oral chloroquine.
3. Angular cheilitis: Inflammaton of corners of mouth.

   Treatment: Correction of predisposing factors. Riboflavin orally.
4. Cheilitis exfoliativa, (Exfoliative cheilitis)

   Treatment: Topical corticosteroids. Plasma cell cheilitis.
5. It resembles Zoon's plasma cell balanitis.

   Treatment: Topical or intralesional steroids.
6. Granulomatosa, swelling and diffuse enlargement of lower lip cheilitis.

   Treatment: Surgical excision, clofazimine.

13. CHLAMYDIA

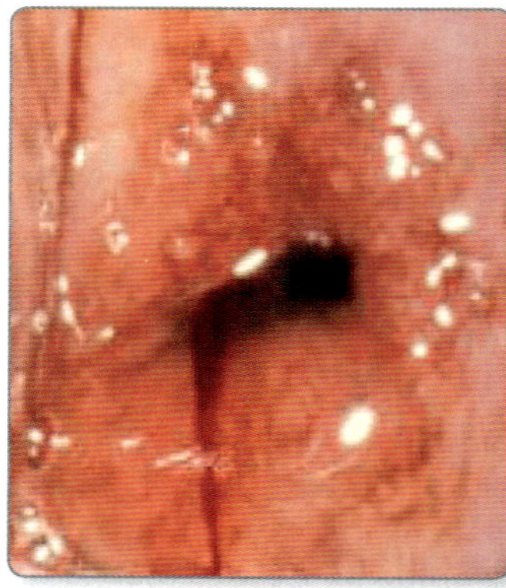

Chlamydia

A sexually transmitted disease (STD) caused by *Chlamydia trachomatis*, or simply chlamydia, a bacterial infection usually infects the genitals of both men and women.

Treatment: Doxycycline 100 mg 2–3 times a day for 10–14 days, or Zithromax® (Azithromycin) 1.0 g (4 x 250 mg) a single dose.

14. CONTACT DERMATITIS

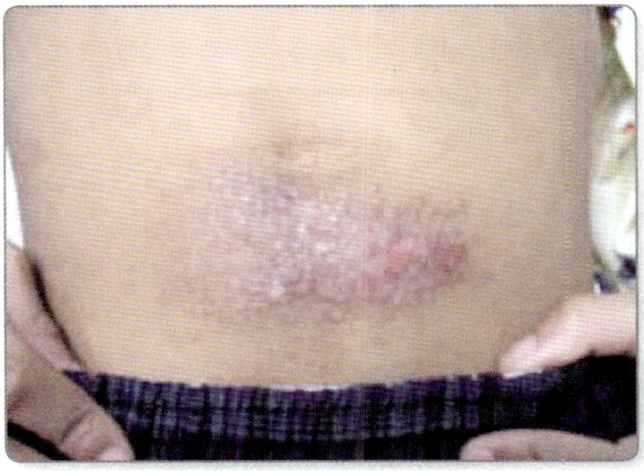

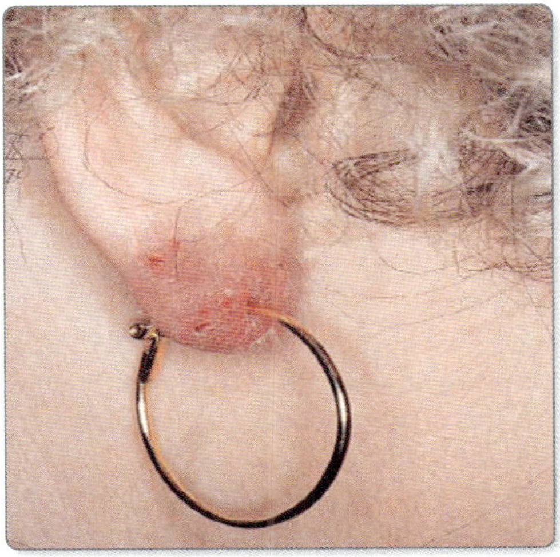

Contact dermatitis

Contact dermatitis is a localized rash or irritation of the skin caused by contact with a foreign substance.

Contact dermatitis is an inflammatory response of the skin to an exogenous substance (irritant and/or allergen). It may be classified as follows:

1. Irritant contact dermatitis (ICD)
   (a) Acute irritant dermatitis
   (b) Cumulative insult dermatitis
2. Allergic contact dermatitis (ACD)
3. Contact urticaria
4. Photo contact dermatitis.

Allergic contact dermatitis (ACD) result when a substance comes into contact with skin which has undergone and acquired specific alteration in its reactivity. This altered reactivity is the result of prior exposure of the skin to the substance.

TYPES OF CONTACT DERMATITIS

Any rash resulting from a substance touching the skin can cause dermatitis by both allergic and non-allergic mechanism. When allergic machanism is involved, it is called allergic contact dermtitis (ACD) and when a non-allergic mechanism is involved and chemically damages the skin, it is called irritant contact dermatitis (ICD).

PATHOMECHANICS, HISTOLOGIC AND CLINICAL EVALUATION OF ACD

Allergic contact dermatitis is an inflammatory reaction mediated by type IV hypersensitivity, i.e. contact sensitivity.

Almost all the allergens that induce and elicit ACD have relatively low molecular weight and belong to hapten immunologically. The skin and its regional lymph nodes play an important role in induction and elicitation of ACD.

Langerhans' cells are the antigen processing and antigen presenting cells. In the regional lymph nodes Langerhans' cells are found mainly in the paracortinal region. The antigen carrying Langerhans' cells encounter with T lymphocytes, react with them and induce an immunoproliferative reaction resulting in a significant increase in circulating sensitized T lymphyocytes which gradually accumulated at the site of challenge and release various lymphokines.

Due to release of various inflammatory mediator substances vascular dilation with edema, and monocellular infiltrate occurs in the upper dermis. This infiltrate extends into the spongiotic epidermis. More and more intercellular edema (Spongiosis) and intracellular edema form in the epidermis. The sequence of inflammatory changes in the dermis and intra- and inter-cellular edema in the epidermis clinically manifest as erythema, swelling, papules which constitute the primary signs of ACD. The usual symptom is intense itching. If contact dermatitis persists because of continued or repeated exposure, the state is set for a subacute or chronic dermatitis.

DIAGNOSIS AND DIFFERENTIAL DIAGNOSIS

The diagnosis of contact dermatitis is based on careful history with a knowledge of common allergens and irritants in the environment. The lesions of ACD can mimic almost any type of eczematous eruption. A selective and probing history and physical examination are essential and should be confirmed by patch testing.

The chief differential diagnosis includes the other eczematous rashes, irritant dermatitis, endogeneous dermatitis (atrophic, eczema, seborrheic eczema, nummular eczema) mycotic infections, psoriasis.

MANAGEMENT

Management of a patient with ACD is aimed mainly at suppression of the skin eruption and prevention of further allergen contact. Corticosteroids are the main stay of treatment. Systemic corticosteroids and topical corticosteriods help a lot. It is possible to replace allergens in an industrial set up; proper protective measures such as cleaning, barrier creams, protective clothing, and gloves and improved ventilation may be useful.

15. CORN

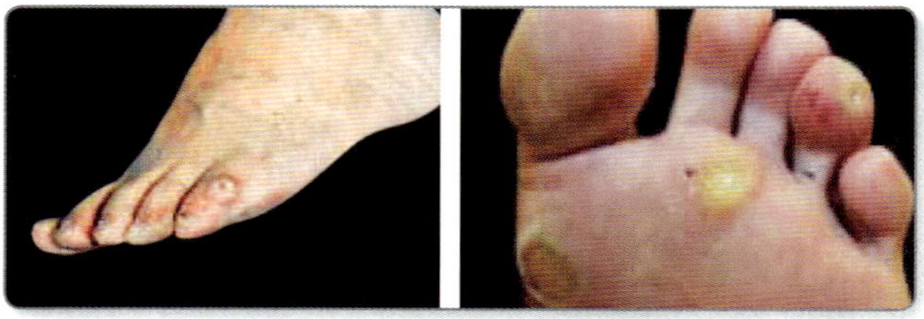

Corn

A 'Corn', also known as clavus is a circumscribed cone-shaped hyperkeratosia of the skin. Its size varies from 1–2 mm upto 2 cm in diameter. The apex of this conical keratotic mass is pointed inwards and presses upon the subjacent structures. Pressure on nerves causes severe pain, especially while walking.

Treatment: Keratolytics

16. CREEPING ERUPTION

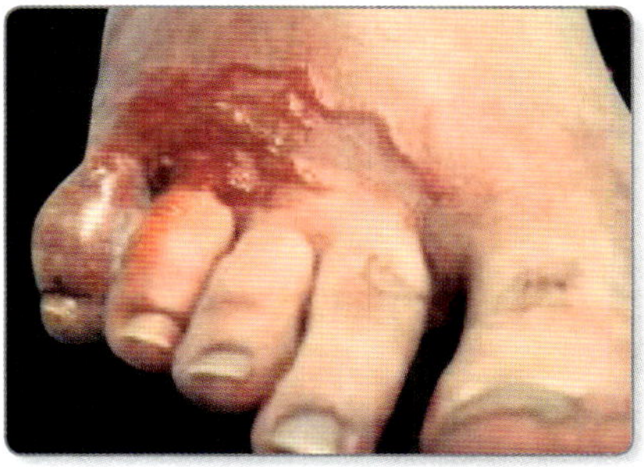

Creeping eruption

Tortuous migratory lesion of the skin caused by burrowing of larvae seen in tropics. The causative organisms are:

1. Larva migrans. Ankylostoma braziliense (cat hookworm), A. caninum (dog hookworm), Uncinaira stenocephala (European dog hookworm), A. ceylonicum, Gnathostoma spinigerum, Bubostomum plebotomum, Dirofilaria capillaria.
2. Larva currens, *Strongyloides stercoralis*.
3. Migratory myiasis, Hypoderma (cattle warble fly), Gastrophilus (horse botfly). Larva migrans is found through hot and humid tropics especially in sandy beaches. Larva penetrates human skin and being unable to complete their life cycle, wander, aimlessly in the lower epidermis.

CLINICAL FEATURES

Feet, hands, buttocks, abdominal wall, commonly affected, scratching, secondary infection, eczema. Self-limiting disease since larvae die in 2–8 weeks. Diagnosis by clinical appearance of typical serpiginous cutaneous lesion with history of exposure to animal excreta.

Treatment: Freezing agents, like liquid nitrogen, ethyl chloride spray over head of the progressive burrow. Local application of 10% thiobendazole solution with steroid cream under occlusion. Oral thiobendazole 50 g/kg body weight, twice daily for two days."Albendazole 400 mg for 3 days.

17. DARIER'S DISEASE

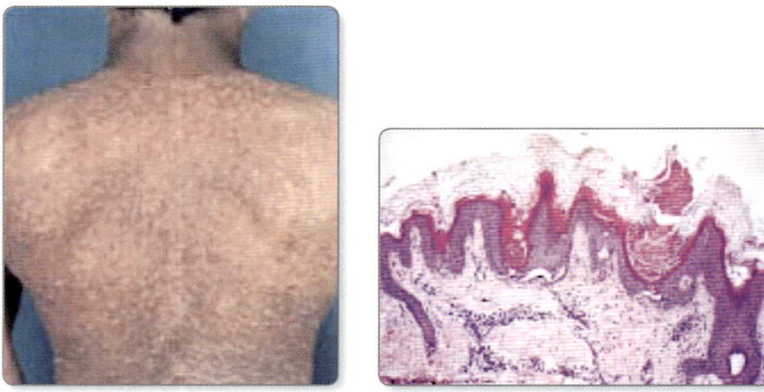

Darier's disease

Darier's disease (DAR), also known as Darier-White disease, dyskeratosis follicularis and keratosis follicularis genetic disorder. Autosomal dominant. From childhood flare occur with heat and humidity. Photosensitivity. Multiple, dirty, warty, papules, symmetrically involving the face, trunks and flexures of the limbs. Seborrheic areas like the neck, shoulders, face, chest; a small pit like depression is seen at the summit of the papule. Palmoplantar pits.

Acrokeratosis verruciformis is a forme fruste of Darier's disease. White cobblestone like papules may be seen on the palate and tongue. Nail changes—longitudinal subungual red and white streaks with subungual keratosis. Cystic changes in the bones. Viruses like herpes simplex and vaccinia cause eczema vaccinatum and eczema herpeticum.

HISTOPATHOLOGY

Hyperkeratosis, acanthosis and papillomatosis, dyskeratosis results in corp ronds and grains. Suprabasal acantholysis leading to formation of suprabasal lacunae.

Treatment: Oral vitinoids topical keratolytics.

18. DERMAL LEISHMANIASIS (DELHI BOIL)

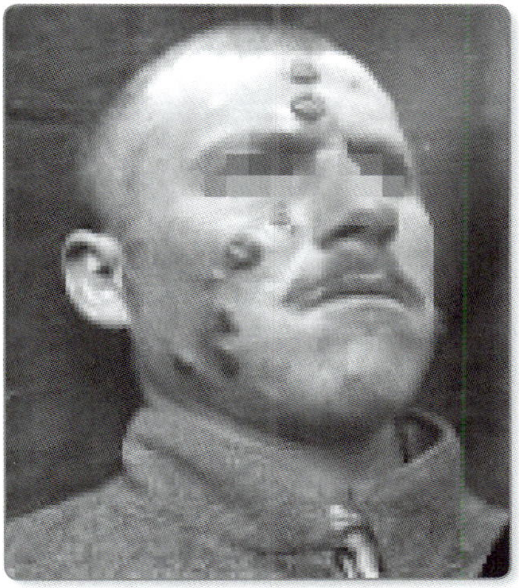

Dermal leishmaniasis (Delhi boil)

Parasitic infection by *Leishmania tropica* transmitted by phlebotomus sandfly.

1. Acute cutaneous leishmaniasis (face, hands): Erythematous, papules like insect bite which ulcerates.
2. Chronic cutaneous leishmaniasis: Papules, nodules, plaques, confirmed by demonstration of Leishman-Donovan (LD) bodies.

Treatment: Pentavalent antimonial preparations, sodium stibogluconate ketaconazole, rifampicin, dapsone, metronidazole, potassium iodide.

19. DERMATITIS HERPETIFORMIS

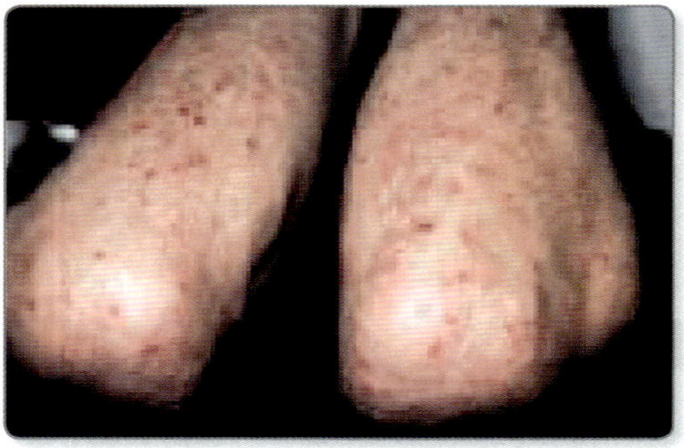

Dematitis herpetiformis

During described this condition in 1884. Usual site shoulders, lumbosacral regions, and elbow. Men are more affected than women.

A gluten sensitive enteropathy present. A chronic blistering skin disease clinically presenting with symmetrical, pleomorphic, intensely pruritic, grouped vesicles arising on an erythematous base. Granular IgA deposit in the dermal papillae on direct immunofluorescence.

Treatment: Dapsone

20. DRUG ERUPTION

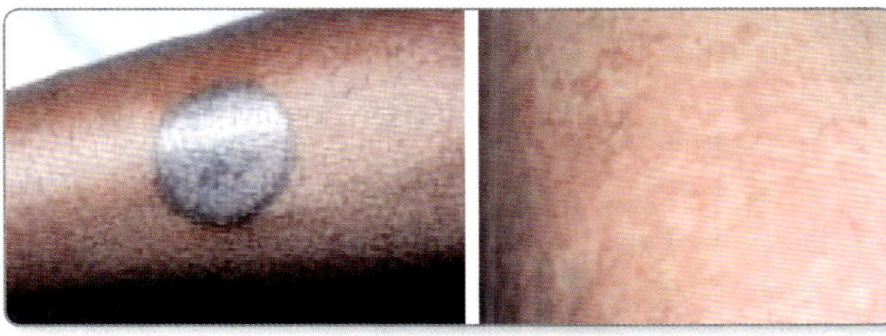

Drug eruption

Drug is a chemical substance or a combination of substances ingested, injected, inhaled, inserted, instilled or topically applied to the skin or mucous membranes for the prevention or treatment of disease.

Clinical patterns of cutaneous drug eruption:

Anaphylaxis
Urticaria and angioedema
Serum sickness
Exanthematous eruption
Fixed drug eruption
Exfoliative dermatitis
Erythema multiforme
Stevens-Johnson syndrome
Toxic epidermal necrolysis
Erythema nodosum
Acneiform eruption
Lichen planus-like eruption
Drug-induced pemphigus
Drug-induced bullous pemphigoid
Iododerma and bromoderma
Purpura
SLE-like syndrome
Scleroderma-like reaction
Photosensitivity
Pigmentary changes
Vasculitis
Pruritus
Acanthosis nigricans
Ichthyosis

DRUG CAUSING ERYTHEMA MULTIFORME

Systemic drugs
Isoniazid
Para-aminosalicylic acid (PAS)

DRUGS CAUSING AN ACNEIFORM ERUPTION

Corticosteroids
Vitamin B12
Oral contraceptives
Androgens
Iodides
Isoniazid
Lithium
Quinidine

DRUGS CAUSING LICHEN PLANUS-LIKE ERUPTION

Chloroquine
Mepacrine
Isoniazid
PAS
Quinidine
Gold
Bismuth
Methyldopa
Propranolol

DRUGS CAUSING A BULLOUS ERUPTION, PEMPHIGUS AND BULLOUS PEMPHIGOID

Drug-induced pemphigus
Penicillin
Ampicillin
Rifampicin
Propranolol
Pemphigoid
Frusemide

DRUGS CAUSING SLE-LIKE SYNDROME

D-penicillamine
Oral contraceptives
Griseofulvin
Isoniazid
Lithium

Treatment: Elimination of the offering drugs. Corticosteroids and antihistamine.

21. ECTHYMA

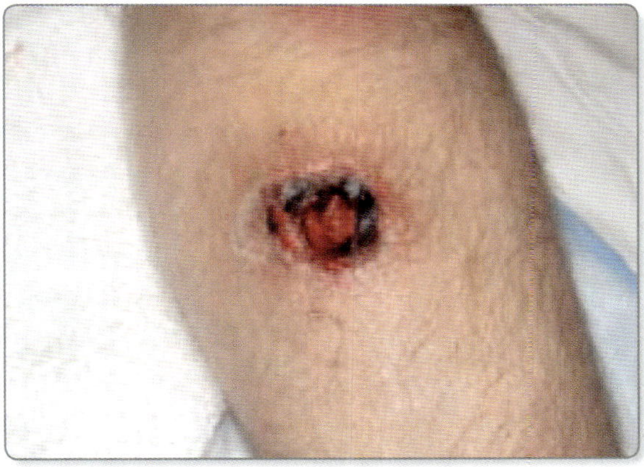

Ecthyma

Deep seated impetigo with thick crust surrounding erythema. The crust is adherent and covering ulcer; healing occurs with scarring. Agent: *Staphylococcus* and *Streptococcus*.

Poor hygiene and malnutrition and repeated trauma are some predisposing factors.

Treatment: Topical and systemic antibiotics.

22. ECZEMA

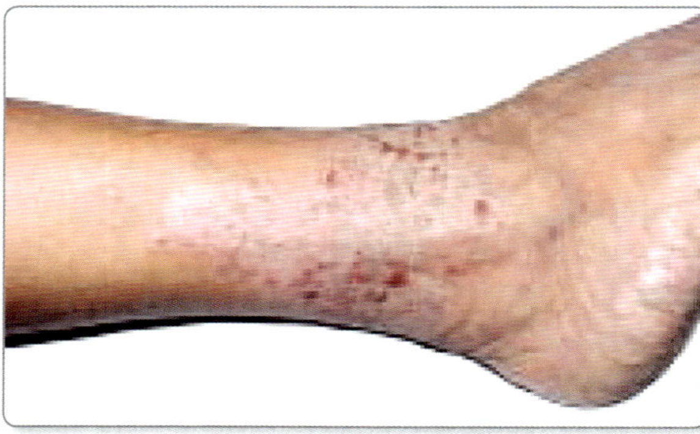

Eczema

Catarrhal inflammation of skin. The term eczema means 'boil out'. Clinically pruritus, erythema, edema, papules, vesicles, scaling and lichenification. Three stages are acute, subacute and chronic.

HISTOPATHOLOGY

Acute: Spongiosis
Subacute: Acanthosis, porokeratosis
Chronic: Hyperkeratosis, acanthosis
Classification of Eczema:

ENDOGENOUS	EXOGENOUS
Atopic dermatitis	Contact dermatitis
Seborrheic dermatitis	Primary irritant dermatitis
Asteatotic eczema	Allergic contact dermatitis
Nummular eczema	Infective eczema
Pityriasis alba	
Stasis dermatitis	
Pompholyx	

Treatment: According to stages oral antihistamine antibiotics if there is secondary infection, corticosteroids in selected cases.

Topical: Corticosteroid creams.

23. ERYTHEMA MULTIFORME

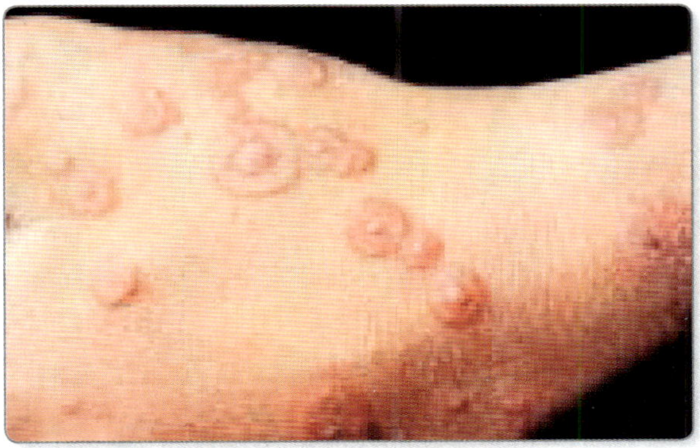

Erythema multiforme

Erythema multiforme is a skin condition of unknown cause, possibly mediated by deposition of immune complex (mostly IgM) in the superficial microvasculature of the skin and oral mucous membrane that usually follows an infection or drug exposure.

Acute self-limiting mucocutaneous condition characterized by multiform lesions: macule, papule, vesicle and bullae and the target lesions or iris lesion.

CAUSATIVE FACTORS

Infection, diseases, drugs, miscellaneous.

INFECTION

Bacterial	Viral	Protozoa	Fungal
1. Streptococcal infection	Herpes simplex	Trichomoniasis	Histoplasmosis Coccidioidomycosis
2. Tuberculosis	Mononucleosis		
3. Syphilis	Orf		
4. Mycoplasma			

Disease	Drug	Miscellaneous
1. Lymphoma	Sulfonamides	Menstruation
2. Leukemia	Penicillin	Pregnancy
		Tetracycline

CLINICAL FEATURES

1. Mild form
2. Severe bullous form sometime fatal called Stevens-Johnson syndrome, malaise, fever, headache, burning at the site, macule, papule and bullae. Oral lesions, ocular lesions present.

DIFFERENTIAL DIAGNOSIS

Bullous pemphigoid, pemphigus vulgaris, erosive lichen planus, Behcet's syndrome, recurrent aphthous ulcers and primary herpetic gingivostomatitis.

Treatment: Oral/Parenteral steroids, antihistamines supportive and symptomatic care. Treatment according to the cause.

24. ERYTHEMA NODOSUM

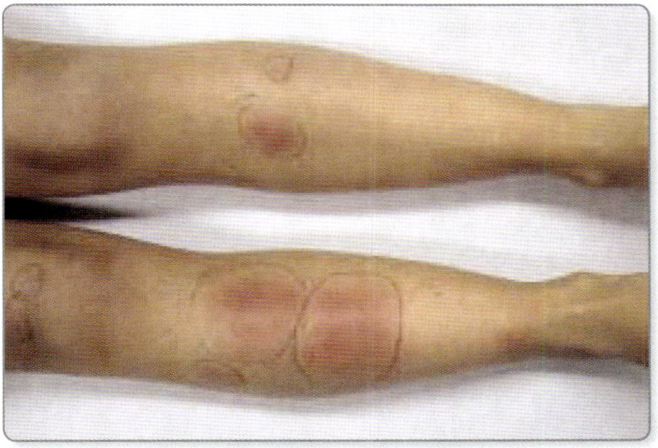

Erythema nodosum

Tender erythematous nodular eruption over extensor aspect of the legs, thighs and forearms. It is a reaction pattern of the skin and allergic in nature.

Weakness, malaise, headache, arthralgia and moderate fever with acute onset of the disease.

HISTOPATHOLOGY

Vasculitis; septal panniculitis.

ETIOLOGY

Infection

Tuberculosis, streptococcal infection, lymphogranuloma venereum, leprosy, cat scratch disease.

Coccidiomycosis, histoplasmosis, blastomycosis, toxoplasmosis, psittacosis, paravaccina infection, dermatophytosis, Milker's nodules, infecion mononucleosis, hepatitis B, and leptospirosis.

DRUGS

Oral contraceptives, sulfonamides, penicillin

COLITIS

Ulcerative colitis

MISCELLANEOUS

Sarcoidosis, Behcet's syndrome, leukemia, Hodgkin's disease

IDIOPATHIC

Investigations

TC, DC, ESR, Mantoux, blood VDRL, X-ray chest, ASO titer, throat culture, Kveim test, skin test with candida, histoplasmin and skin biopsy.

COURSE

Spontaneous healing in about 3–6 weeks

Treatment: The best treatment is to eradicate the underlying cause, rest, potassium iodide, corticosteroids, antibiotics, colchicine.

25. EXFOLIATIVE DERMATITIS

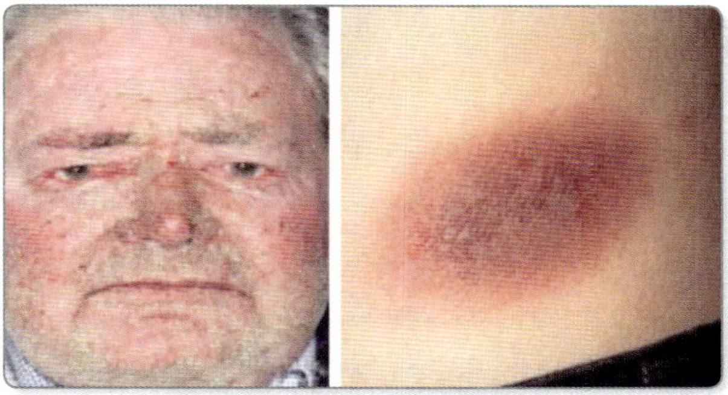

Exfoliative dermatitis

Universal desquamation and erythema with thickening of the skin. Exfoliation may be slight but erythema is generally universal.

Etiology of Exfoliative Dermatitis		
Existing skin disease	**Systematic disease**	**Drugs**
Atopic dermatitis	Acute leukemia	Arsenic
Contact dermatitis	Hodgkin's diseases	Aspirin
Dermatophytosis	Lymphoma	Chloroquine
Eczema	Mycosis fungoides	Dapsone
Ichthyosis		Cold
Lichen planus		
Pemphigus foliaceus		
Psoriasis		
Reiter's syndrome		

Males are affected two to three times more frequently than females.

PATHOGENESIS

The universal redness of the skin and scaling due to alteration in keratinization. This vasodilation may lead to high-output cardiac failure, thermoregulatory control failure and the patient becomes poikilothermic. Critical losses of water, proteins and electrolytes occur. There may be hypoalbuminemia and edema of the feet. There is an increase in the rate of epidermal turnover which leads to continuous exfoliation. There is negative nitrogen balance and a negative potassium balance. The changes in blood are anemia (due to iron loss) eosinophilia, leukocytosis, peripheral blood-lymphocytosis, serum electrolyte abnormalities, elevated ESR.

SYSTEMIC MANIFESTATION

Hepatomegaly and splenomegaly. The basal metabolic rate is raised.

PROGNOSIS

Depends upon underlying cause.

Treatment: General measures, treatment of underlying causes, good nursing care, antibiotic, steroid, antihistamine immunosuppressives.

26. FIXED DRUG ERUPTION

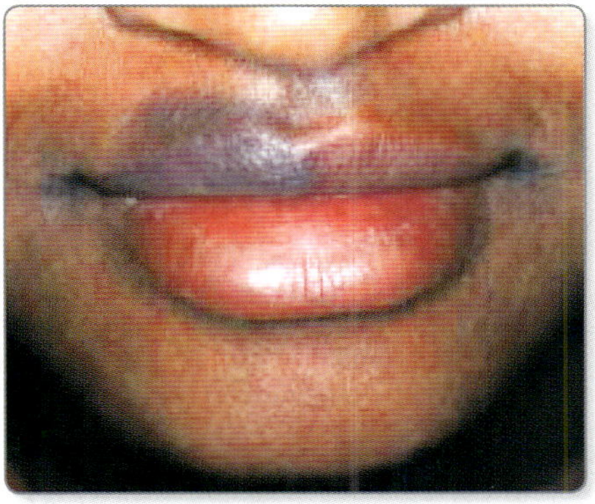

Fixed drug eruption

It occurs at the same site following the administration of any offending drug. Clinically it may be oval, well-marginated, erythematous, violaceous or hyperpigmented lesion. Any part of the body is affected but frequently oral mucosa and glans penis is inolved.

DRUGS CAUSING FIXED DRUG ERUPTION

Sulfonamides
Salicylates
Oxyphenbutazone
Tetracycline
Dapsone
Phenolphthalein
Morphine
Codeine
Quinine and derivatives

Treatment: Avoid further intake of offending drugs. Topical corticosteroids and systemic corticosteroids and antihistamine.

27. FRECKLES

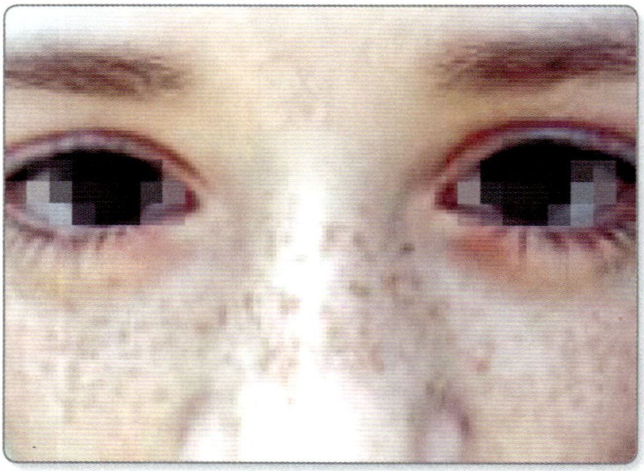

Freckles

Small circumscribed pale brown macules (less than 5 mm) over face especially sun exposed area. More in summer.

Treatment: Sunscreening agents. Depigmenting agents - Hydroquinone, steroids, retinoic acid.

28. FUNGUS DERMATOPHYTOSES

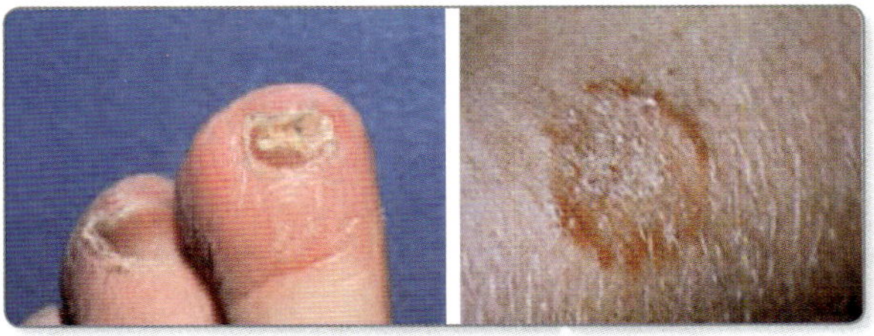

Fungus dermatophytoses

A superficial fungal infection of keratinized tissue caused by dermatophytes.

Three important genera: Microsporum, Trichophyton and Epidermophyton. They may be geophilic, zoophilic or anthropophilic.

	Clinical types	Area	Organisms
1.	Tinea capitis	Scalp	*T. violaceum,* *T. rubrum,* *T. mentagrophytes*
2.	Tinea barbae	Beard	*T. mentagrophytes* *T. verrucosum*
3.	Tinea corporis and limbs	Glabrous trunk	*T. rubrum,* *M. canis*
4.	Tinea pedis	Groin, perineum, perianal region	*Epidermophyton floccosum,* *Trichophyton*
5.	Tinea pedis	Feet	*T. mentagrophytes,* *T. rubrum*
6.	Tinea manuum	Hands	
7.	Tinea unguium (Onychomycosis)	Nail	*T. rubrum*
8.	Tinea faciei	Face	*T. rubrum*
9.	Tinea incognito (Steroid modified tinea)		

PREDISPOSING FACTORS

Poor nutrition, unhygienic conditions, hot and humid climate, sweating and maceration, diabetes mellitus, debilitating diseases, corticosteroids and immunosuppressive therapy.

1. Tinea capitis
   Infection transmitted through combs, hairbrushes, and hats. Gray patch, black dot, seborrheic variety, kerion, alopecia areata like, favus.
2. Tinea barbae
   Ringworm infection of the beard and moustache areas of the face.
3. Tinea corporis
   Infection of the glabrous skin, classical ringworm starts as erythematous, itchy papule which progresses to form a circinate lesion. The periphery is studded with papules and papulovesicles.
4. Tinea cruris
   Ringworm infection localized to the groin, perineum and perianal region.
5. Tinea pedis
   Ringworm of the feet, manifesting as hyperkeratoic lesion, intertriginous lesion, vesicular and bullous lesions.
6. Tinea manuum
   Superficial fungal infection of the hands.
7. Tinea unguium (Onychomycosis)
   Ringworm infection of the nails.
8. Tinea faciei
   Superficial ringworm infection of the face.
9. Tinea incognito: Steroid modified tinea

Treatment: Systemic griseofulvin or ketaconazole. Topical imidazole derivatives, Whitfield's ointment.

LABORATORY DIAGNOSIS

1. Potassium hydroxide (KOH) examination of scales
2. Examination of the blister roof
3. Culture on Sabouraud's media with cycloheximide and chloramphenicol
4. Wood's lamp examination
5. Biopsy with PAS stain

29. FURUNCULOSIS

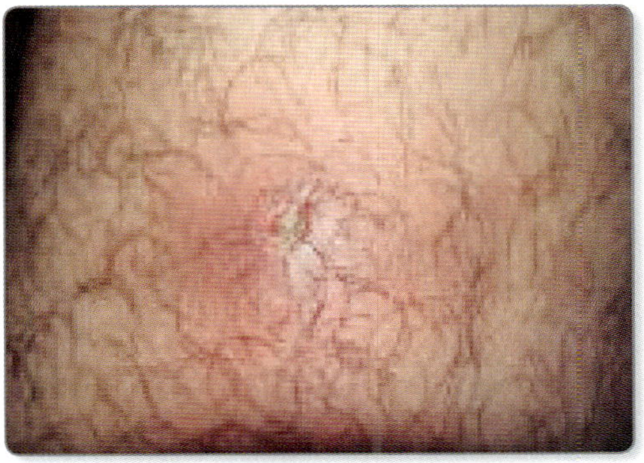

Furunculosis

Folliculitis is the inflammation of one or more hair follicles. Caused by *Staphylococcus aureus*, inflammation of the hair-follicle including perifollicular region in the dermis and subcutaneous tissue. Precipitation factors like diabetes mellitus and systemic steroids.

Treatment: Antibiotics.

30. GONORRHEA

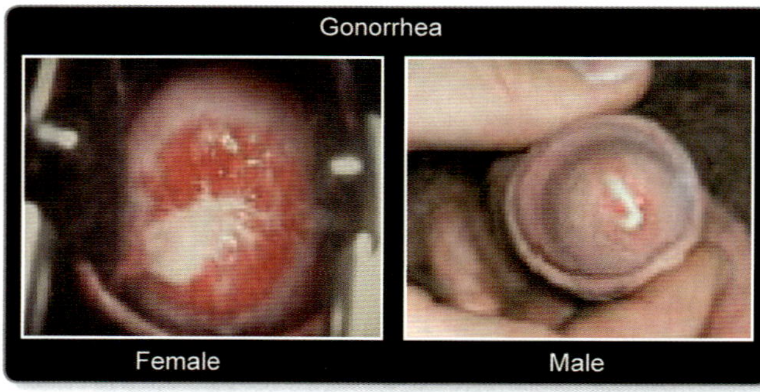

Gonorrhea

A highly contagious sexually transmitted bacterial infection. Caused by *Neisseria gonorrhoeae*. Characterized by thick discharge from the penis or vagina. Gonorrhea may infect the rectum, throat, eyes, blood, skin, and joints. Gonorrhea spreads through semen or vaginal fluids during unprotected sexual contact, heterosexual or homosexual, with an infected partner. Gonorrhea incubation period is 1–14 days. A urine test and a swab test confirm the diagnosis. "Infections due to *Neisseria gonorrhoeae*, like those due to *Chlamydia trachomatis*, remain a major cause of pelvic inflammatory disease, tubal infertility, ectopic pregnancy, and chronic pelvic pain.

Treatment: Cefixime 400 mg orally in a single dose.

Ceftriaxone 125 mg IM in a single dose, ciprofloxacin 500 mg orally in a single dose, ofloxacin 400 mg orally in a single dose plus azithromycin 1 g orally in a single dose, doxycycline 100 mg orally twice a day for 7 days.

31. GRANULOMA ANNULARE

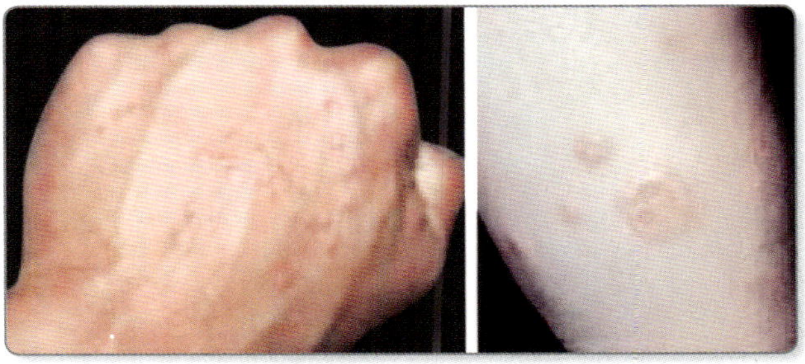

Granuloma annulare

Numerous skin colored papules often symmetrically distributed and they are either discrete of coalesce to form small plaques in annulare or reticulate patterns. Lesions of subcutaneous nodules. Corticosteroids such as clobetasol propionate or methylprednisolone. Subdermally injected corticosteroids such as triamcinolone have also been effective in reducing the size and spread of granuloma annulare. Granuloma annulare is a marker of diabetes mellitus in adults. Treatment may not be necessary except for cosmetic reasons.

DIFFERENTIAL DIAGNOSIS

Gumma ringworm, syphilid, tuberculid, lymphoma cutis and sarcoidosis.

32. GRANULOMA PYOGENICUM
(SYN. GRANULOMA TELANGIECTATICUM)

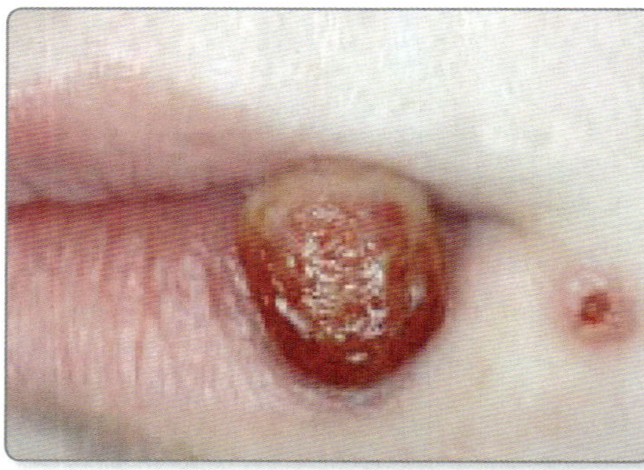

Granuloma pyogenicum

CLINICAL FEATURES

It is usually solitary and seen in both sexes in any age. Solitary granuloma pyogenicum is frequently located on the face and scalp. The tumor consists of a dark red, soft or moderately firm, raised or pedunculated nodule; it bleeds easily when traumatized.

PATHOLOGY

Granuloma pyogenicum shows a lobulated arrangement with endothelial proliferation.

Treatment: Complete removal by surgical excision. Curettage and cauterization, by diathermy, cryotherapy and laser.

33. HANSEN'S DISEASE

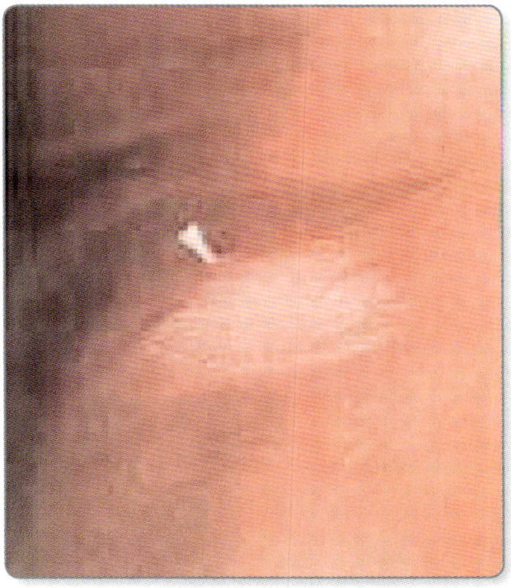

Tuberculoid leprosy

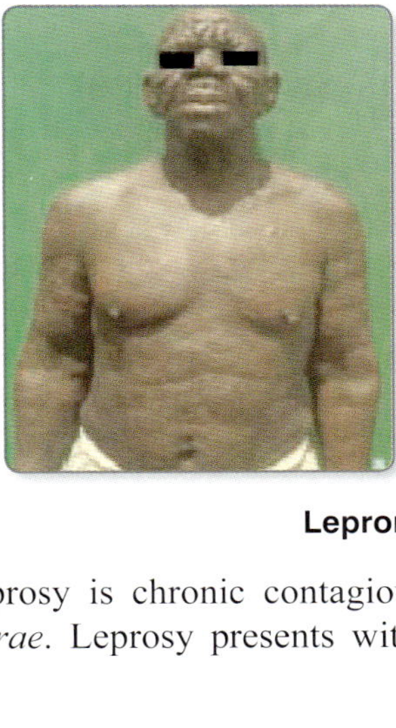

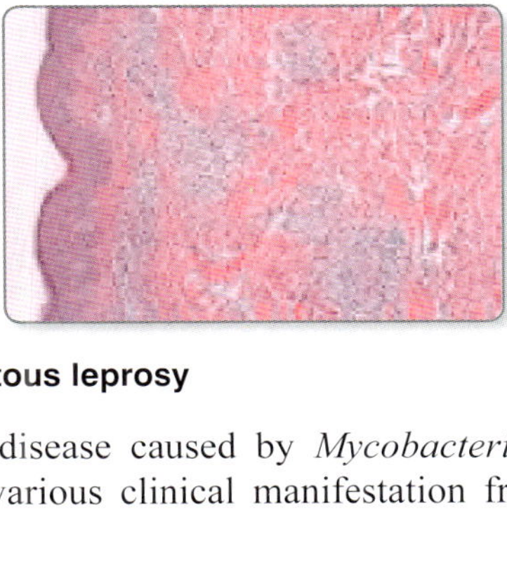

Lepromatous leprosy

Leprosy is chronic contagious disease caused by *Mycobacterium leprae*. Leprosy presents with various clinical manifestation from an insignificant skin lesion to extensive disease causing profound disability and disfigurement by damaging peripheral nerve eyes, bones other tissues. Three cardinal diagnostic features of leprosy are:

1. Finding acid fast bacilli in skin or nose
2. Sensory changes of the skin
3. Thickening of the nerves.

Riley-Jopling Classification	
TT	Tuberculoid leprosy
BT	Borderline tuberculoid
BB	Midborderline leprosy
BL	Borderline lepramatous
LL	Lepromatous leprosy

TUBERCULOID LEPROSY

- Clinically by neural and skin involvement
- Bacteriologically few or no bacilli in the lesion
- Histologically by tuberculoid reaction
- Immunologically by high cell-mediated immunity manifested by positive lepromin test.

LEPROMATOUS LEPROSY

Leprosy or Hansen's disease (HD) is a chronic disease caused by the bacteria *Mycobacterium leprae* and *Mycobacterium lepromatosis*. Named after physician Gerhard Armauer Hansen, leprosy is primarily a granulomatous disease of the peripheral nerves and mucosa of the upper respiratory tract; skin lesions are the primary external sign.

Clinically by skin lessions, macules, diffuse infiltration, nodules, mucosal changes and late neural and systemic involvement.

Bacteriologically plenty of bacilli in the lesions.

Histologically by granulomatous infiltrate containing lepra cells.

Immunologically by negative lepromin test with absence of cell-mediated immunity.

INDETERMINATE LEPROSY

- Clinically by hypopigmented macules and neural involvement
- Bacteriologically no bacilli or few

- Histologically nonspecific inflammatory reaction
- Immunologically variable response to lepromin test

LEPRA REACTIONS

1. Type 1 lepra reaction (Acute exacerbation) upgrading and dowgrading seen in borderline leprosy.

   Treatment: Prednisolone and clofazimine systemic

2. Type 2 lepra reaction (Erythema nodosum leprosum–ENL) seen in lepromatous leprosy.

   Treatment: Antimalarials, thalidomide, corticosteroids, clofazimine.

TREATMENT OF LEPROSY

Dapsone, rifampicin, clofazimine.

34. HERPES SIMPLEX

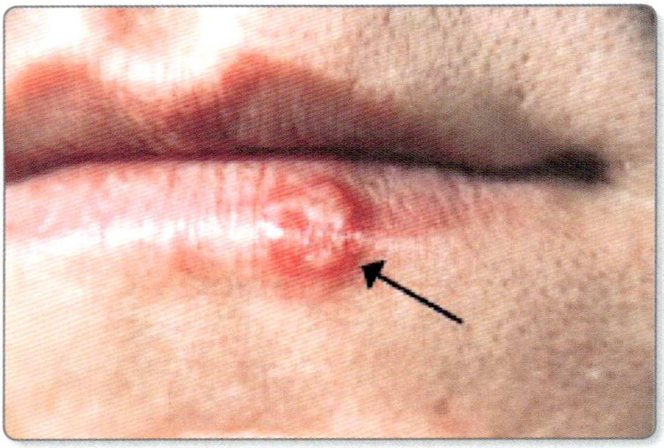

Herpes simplex

Caused by herpes virus hominis type I and type II. Type I affects cutaneous, oropharyngeal, ocular areas. HSV type II affects genital tract.

HISTOPATHOLOGY

Ballooning degeneration, intracellular edema, reticular degeneration, giant cells, viral inclusion bodies.

The clinical entities predominantly caused by HSV type 1 are:

a. Herpetic gingivostomatitis
b. Herpes labialis
c. Herpetic whitlow
d. Eczema herpeticum
e. Zosteriform herpes simplex
f. Ocular herpes simplex
g. Central nervous system (CNS) involvement
h. Disseminated herpes.

Treatment: Genital herpes—Anti-viral agents like acyclovir, idoxyuridine, ribavirin.

ACYCLOVIR

200 mgs tablets of acyclovir can be given 5 times a day for 5 days. Topically acyclovir (5% cream) applied five times daily for five days may be used.

RIBAVIRIN

800 mg orally for 7–10 days.

35. HERPES ZOSTER

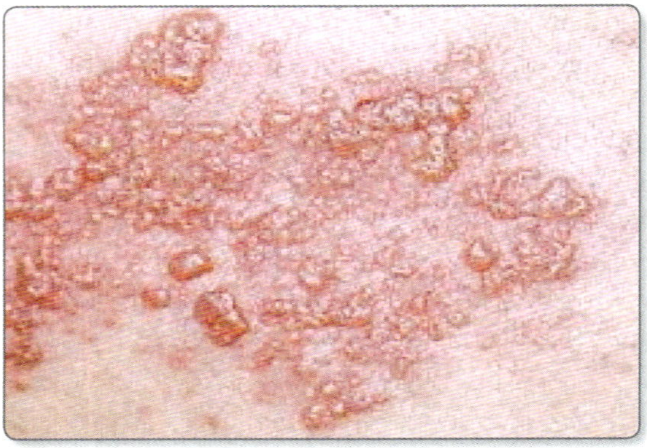

Herpes zoster

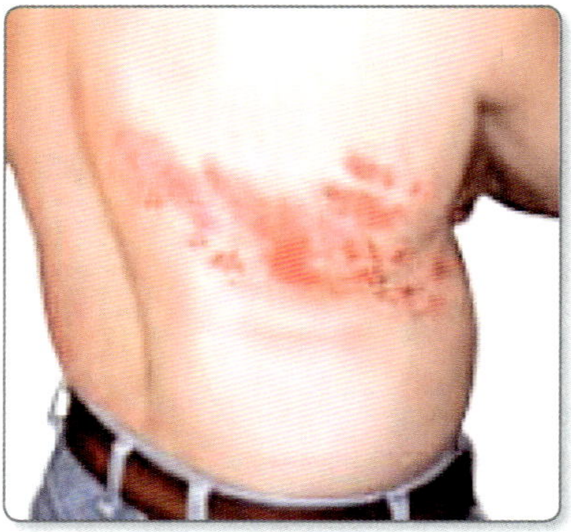

Prodromal symptoms

Herpes zoster (Shingles) is a localized reactivation of the chickenpox virus (varicella-zoster virus) which previously remained dormant in the dorsal root ganglia. This DNA viral disease by nature occurs in a patient who previously suffered from varicella. The causes for reactivation are unknown. Occasionally, harpes zoster is associated with cancer.

PRODROMAL SYMPTOMS

Itching, tingling, burning sensation or pain, in the involved dermatome, tenderness and hyperesthesia of the skin.

The rash: Unilateral and does not cross the midline. Closely grouped, erythematous maculopapules, which rapidly become vesicular in 12 to 24 hours. The regional lymph nodes enlarged and tender. Recovery takes about 3 to 4 weeks or longer in older patients. Complications of herpes zoster:

1. Hypopigmented or hyperpigmented scars
2. Post herpetic neuralgia
3. Post herpetic anesthesia
4. Involvement of motor neurons—motor zoster
5. Ocular complications: Neuroparalytic keratitis with corneal ulceration, panophthalmitis, iritis leading to iris atrophy.
6. Other complications such as encephalomyelitis, meningitis and pneumonitis, zoster-hemiplegia syndrome.

LABORATORY DIAGNOSIS

Tzanck smears, for giant cells skin biopsy, complement fixation, Electron microscopic study.

Treatment: Bed rest, analgesics topically IDU, silver sulfadiazine and acyclovir. Systemic drugs are antibiotics and antivirals. Treatment of post-herptic neuralgia (PHN)–Capsaicin (0.25%) topically, tegretol, phenytoin sodium orally.

36. HYPERHIDROSIS

Hyperhidrosis is excessive sweating. Hyperhidrosis is broadly classified as, generalized and localized.

INVESTIGATION OF HYPERHIDROSIS

Triggering factors: Emotional, lacrimal, gustatory or spontaneous, diabetic mellitus and other diseases must be ruled out.

Treatment

Systemic: Anticholinergic drug or atropine analogs.

Topical: 10% formaldehyde. 10% glutaraldehyde sympathectomy.

37. ICHTHYOSIS

Ichthyosis means a generalized persistent non-inflammatory scaling disorder of the skin surface.

GENETIC AND ACQUIRED

Genetic

1. Ichthyosis vulgaris
2. X-linked ichthyosis
3. Congenital ichthyosiform erythroderma–Bullous
4. Congenital ichthyosiform erythroderma–Non-bullous
5. Erythrokeratoderma variabilis
6. Ichthyosis linearis circumflexation

Acquired

1. Hypothyroid
2. Hansen's disease
3. Diabetes mellitus
4. Malignancy
5. Drugs

SYNDROMES ASSOCIATED WITH ICHTHYOSIS

1. Sjogren-Larsson syndrome (Mental deficiency, spastic paralysis)
2. Rud's syndrome
3. Refsum syndrome
4. Netherton syndrome.

Treatment: Topical applications emollients like vegetable oil, liquid paraffin, vaseline, propylene glycol, 10% urea.

38. IMPETIGO

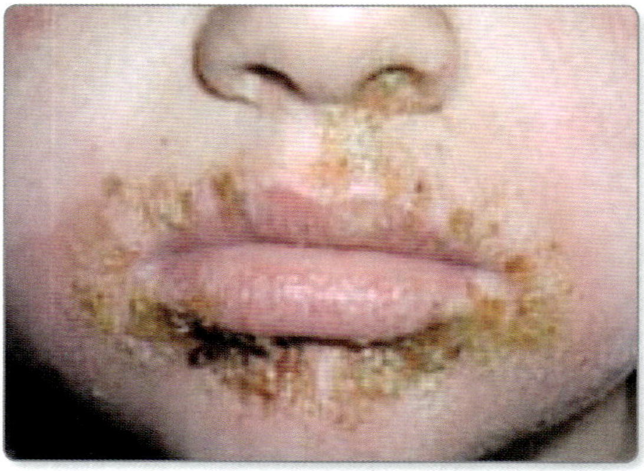

Impetigo

Superficial contagious bacterial infection of the skin. The most common skin infection in children. Impetigo can be divided into the bullous and non-bullous forms caused by *Staphylococcus aureus*, Streptococcus or both.

Infection of the Skin Due to Bacteria		
Disease	**Target tissue**	**Causative organism**
Impetigo	Epidermis	Streptococcus and/or Staphylococcus
Ecthyma	Epidermis	Streptococcus and/or Staphylococcus
	Dermis	Staphylococcus
Erysipelas	Dermis	Streptococcus
Cellulitis	Dermis, subcutaneous tissues	Streptococcus
Folliculitis	Hair follicle (Upper)	Staphylococcus
Furuncle	Hair follicle (Upper+Lower)	Staphylococcus
Carbuncle	Hair follicle (Multiple)	Staphylococcus

It can be primary impetigo or secondary impetigo. Primary impetigo arises from normal skin. Secondary impetigo arises from pre-existing dermatoses (Scabies, pediculosis).

Sudden onset, primary lesion is a thin-walled vesicle which breaks discharging stickly serum. This dries forming honey colored, adherent crusts. If the crust is removed, moist red-eroded area is seen.

Treatment: Topical antibiotic cream and systemic antibiotics.

39. INSECT BITE ALLERGY (PAPULAR URTICARIA)

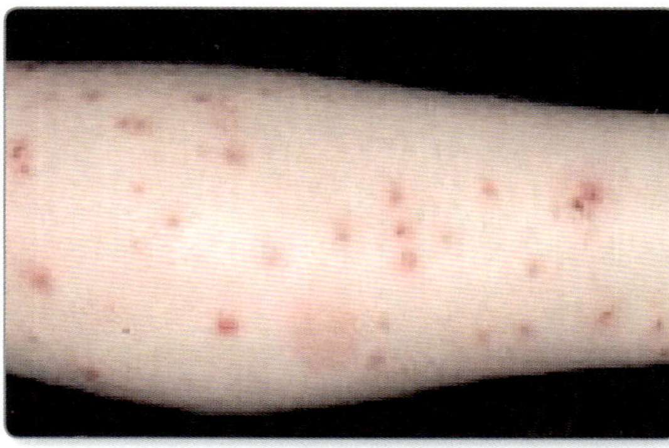

Papular urticaria

Papular urticaria may be defined as a chronic recurrent eruption of irritable urticated papules. Acquired sensitivity to insect bites. The lesions have characteristic distribution and seasonal incidence. Essentially a disease of children. A number of insects other than mosquitoes also cause this. The primary lesions are wheals, and papules. Scratching and secondary infection vesicles, bullae, eczematous plaques, purpuric blotches or thickened patches can be seen.

40. INTERTRIGO

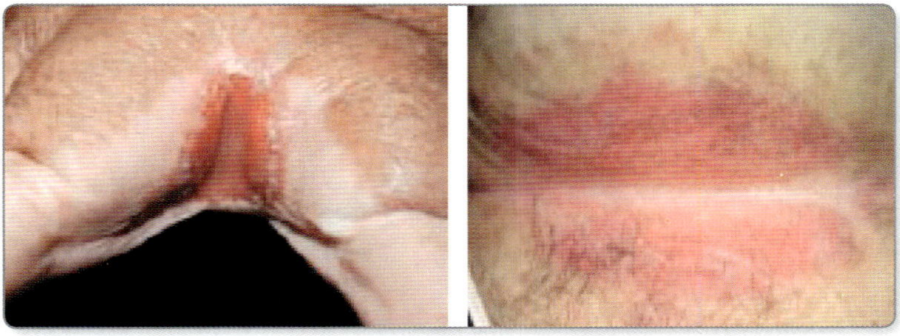

Intertrigo

Intertrigo is an inflammatory dermatoses involving the body folds. Physical factors like friction, moisture and occlusion humid climate (which causes sweating), poor hygiene.

Most adults who have intertrigo are obese, diabetic or both.

The organisms are usually *Staphylococcus aureus*, *Streptococcus pyogenes*, *Streptococcus haemolyticus*, *E. coil*, *Pseudomonas aeruginosa, Candida*.

Well-marginated erythema confined to the areas of skin apposition. The axillary, intergluteal, and genitocrural folds are commonly involved.

Treatment: Drying of the area and treatment of secondary bacterial or candidal infection and obesity.

41. KELOID

Keloid (Greek for claw like) and hypertrophic scar are overgrowth of scar tissues within the dermis. Factors influencing their development are:

1. Trauma
2. Skin tension
3. Race: There is prediction for dark-skinned races especially Negroes.

Treatment: Intralesional triamcinolone, cryotherapy.

42. KERION

Tinea capitis suppurative pattern. It is a painful inflammatory mass. Follicles may be seen discharging pus. Lymphadenopathy frequent. Zoophilic fungus or *T. mentagrophytes*. Bacterial co-pathogen present.

Treatment: Griseofulvin and ketaconazole. Antibiotic if secondary infection.

43. LICHEN NITIDUS

Multiple tiny nonpruritic shiny papules with a flat surface appear on the arms, abdomen and penis.

HISTOPATHOLOGY

Infiltrate is just below flattened epidermis and it is well circumscribed. It consists of lymphocytes, histiocytes and a few Langhans giant cells and plasma cells. Claw clutching a ball appearance.

Treatment: It is symptomatic since self-limiting. No treatment is required in most cases.

44. LICHEN PLANUS

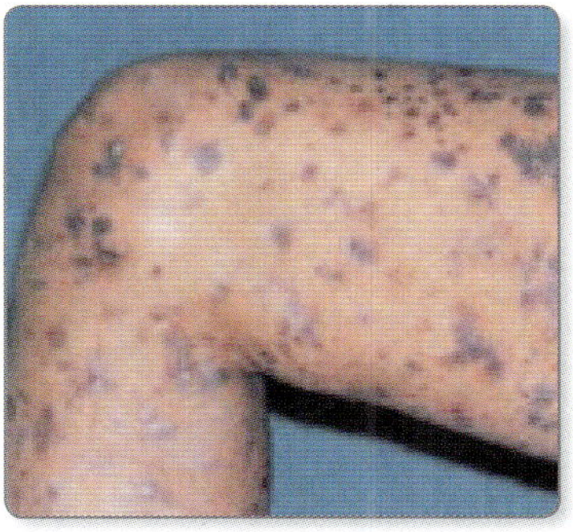

Lichen planus

Lichen planus is usually a self-limited eruption which can involve the skin, mucous membranes, hair and nail.

CLINICAL FEATURES

Violaceous, itchy, polygonal, shiny flat-topped papules. Wickham's striae. The Koebner phenomenon is common.

The types of lichen planus.

Actinic
Annular
Atrophic
Bullous
Classical
Erythematous
Exfoliative
Follicular
Guttate
Hypertrophic
Linear
Mucous membrane
Nail
Oral
Perforating
Pigmentosus
Planopilaris
Ulcerative

PATHOGENESIS

The cause unknown. Infective, psychogenic, genetic and immunological factors are among the etiological factors considered.

COMPLICATIONS

Squamous cell carcinoma (Ulcerative mucosal LP), scarring alopecia, nail dystrophy.

Treatment

Topical steroids	Systemic drug, oral synthetic retinoids chloroquine
Intralesional steroids	Corticosteroids
Phototherapy	Dapsone

45. LICHEN STRIATUS

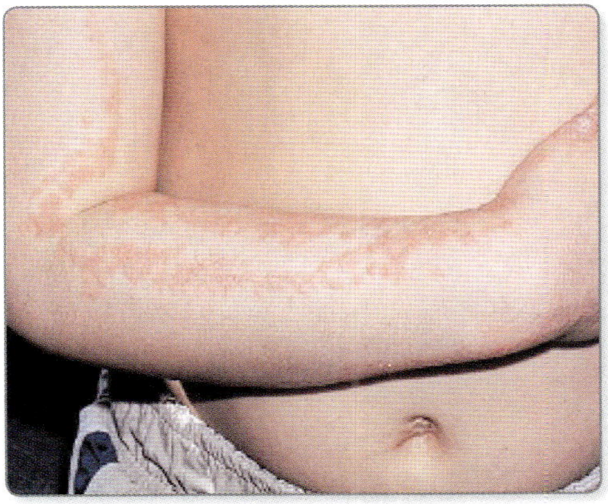

Lichen striatus

It is an acquired self-limiting inflammatory linear disorder of unknown etiology.

CLINICAL FEATURES

Children aged 5–15 years. The linear band of hypopigmented lichenoid papules which tend to coalesce. The lesion commonly occurs on one arm but may be seen elsewhere along Blaschko's lines.

Treatment: Not necessary.

46. LICHENOID REACTION

- Lichen planus-like skin eruption can occur with various drugs and chemicals.
- Drug associated with an LP-like reaction
- Antihypertensives
- Beta blockers paraphenylenediamines (CD-2 and CD-3)
- Methyldopa
- Gold
- Tetracycline
- Streptomycin
- Griseofulvin
- Indomethacin
- Chloroquine
- Quinine

Treatment

The treatment of lichenoid eruption is to withdraw the drug or avoid contact with the chemical.

47. LUPUS ERYTHEMATOSUS

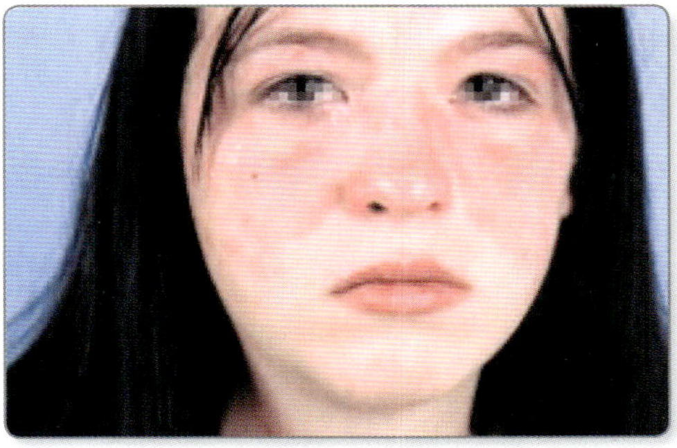

Lupus erythematosus

DISCOID LUPUS ERYTHEMATOSUS

It is a connective tissue discorder of the skin of uncertain etiology. The cutaneous lesions of DLE consist of well defined erythematous, slightly infiltrated discoid patches which show adherent thick scales and follicular plugging.

CLINICAL TYPE

Discoid type, verrucous DLE, tumid type of DLE, lupus erythematous telangiectodes, annular atrophic plaque, chilblain lupus, lupus erythematosis and erythema multiforme-like syndrome (Rowell's syndrome), lupus erythematous profundus (Panniculitis), lupus erythematosus hypertropicus and profundus, rosacea-like DLE.

HISTOPATHOLOGY

- Hyperkeratosis with follicular plugging
- Thinning and flattening of the stratum malpighii
- Hydropic degeneration of basal cells
- A lymphocytic infiltrate which tends to be arranged around the appendages.

- Edema, vasodilation and slight extravasation of erythrocytes in the upper dermis.

Treatment: Topical steroids, sunscreening agents, oral dapsone, chloroquine, thalidomide, clofazimine, oral retinoids.

SYSTEMIC LUPUS ERYTHEMATOSUS

Definition

Systemic lupus erythematosus (SLE) is a connective tissue disorder of unknown etiology in which tissues and cells are damaged by deposition of pathogenic autoantibodies and immune complex.

DIAGNOSIS OF SLE

- Mar rash
- Discoid rash
- Photosensitivity
- Oral or nasopharyngeal ulcers usually painless
- Non-erosive, arthritis
- Serositis (pleurisy or pericarditis)
- Renal disorder (persistent proteinuria exceeding 0.5 g/day, cellular casts)
- Neurologic disorder (seizures or psychosis)
- Hematologic disorders (hemolytic anemia with reticulocytosis leukopenia and lymphopenia of less than 1500/mm or thrombocytopenia less than 100,000/mm)
- Abnormal ANA titer.

Immunologic disorder (positive LE cell reparation, anti-DNA antibody in abnormal titer, antibody to Sm nuclear antigen, or positive test for syphilis known to be false positive for at least six months and confirmed by TPI or FTA-ABS test.

The American Rheumatism Association (ARA) has developed criteria for the diagonosis of SLE. The presence of any four of these or a total of four when combined with certain autoantibodies established a diagnosis of definite SLE.

Treatment: Rest and sunscreen, antimalarials, oral steroids, dapsone immunosuppressive drugs, cyclophosphamide, azathioprine).

48. LUPUS VULGARIS

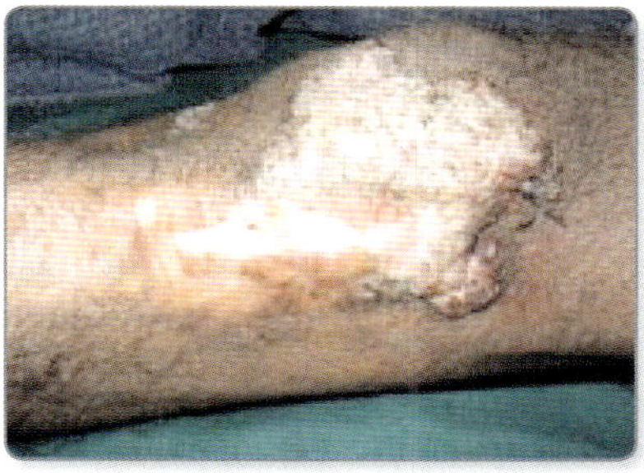

Lupus vulgaris

Common type of cutaneous tuberculosis. Both exogenous and hematogenous spread can occur. Moderate degree of immunity. The initial lesion is erythematous nodule, slightly elevated above the surface, and later coalesce to form a soft plaque.

In the classical description of lupus vulgaris, the presence of apple-jelly nodules at the edge of a plaque is often mentioned. They do not exhibit this color in Indian skin.

The lesion should be differentiated from other granulomata like syphilitic gumma, leprosy, systemic fungal infection, leishmaniasis (lupoid form), sarcoidosis.

CLASSIFICATION OF CUTANEOUS TUBERCULOSIS

Exogenous source	Tuberculosis chancre
	Warty tuberculosis
	Lupus vulgaris
Endogenous source	
Contiguous spread	Scrofuloderma
Auto-inoculation	Orificial tuberculosis
Hematogenous	Lupus vulgaris
	Tuberculosis gumma.

TUBERCULID: A HYPERSENSITIVITY TO THE TB BACILLI

Micropapular	Lichen scrofulosoram
Macropapular	Papular or papulonecrotic tuberculid
Macropapular	Erythema nodosum
Nodular	Erythema induratum (Brain)

49. LYMPHOGRANULOMA VENEREUM (LGV)

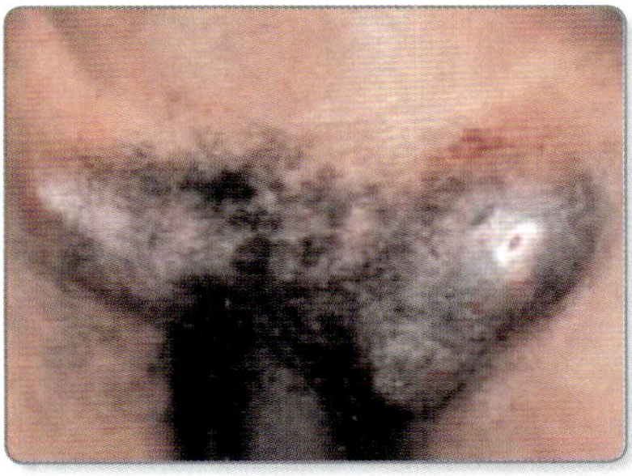

Lymphogranuloma venereum (LGV)

A sexually transmitted bacterial chronic infection caused by *Chlamydia trachomatis*.

More common in men than women. More risk factor is being HIV-positive. Clinically an oozing, abnormal connection (fistula) in the rectal area, a sore on the genitals, drainage through the skin from lymph nodes in the groin, swelling of the vulva or labia in women, swollen lymph nodes in the groin (inguinal lymphadenopathy). Confirmation of the diagnosis includes biopsy of the lymph node, blood test for the bacteria that causes LGV, laboratory test to detect Chlamydia.

Treatment: This condition is cured with the right antibiotics. Antibiotics that are commonly prescribed to treat LGV include tetracycline, doxycycline, erythromycin, and azithromycin.

50. MACULAR ATROPHY

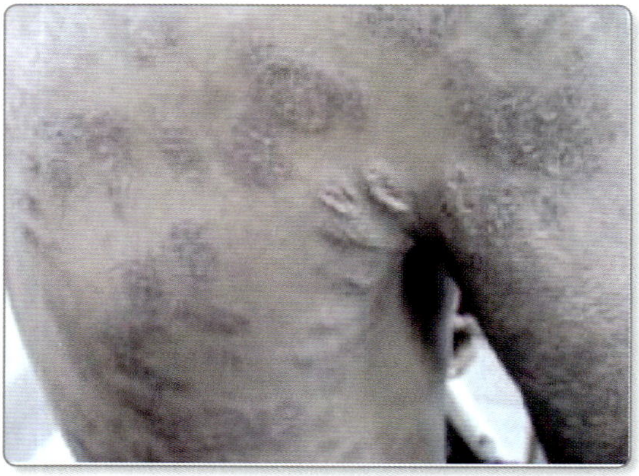

Macular atrophy

Macular atrophy or anetoderma: Atrophic patch located mainly over the upper trunk. Two types: One Jadassohn type (Inflammatory type) and Schweninger-Buzzi type (non-inflammatory type). Secondary macular atrophy occurs after various diseases like syphilis, lupus erythematosus and leprosy.

51. MILIARIA

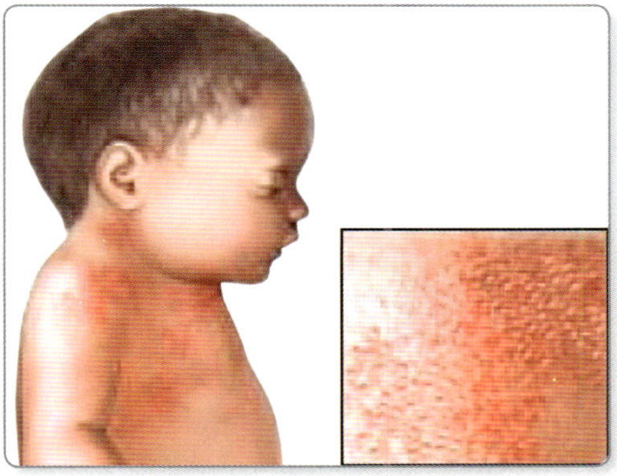

Miliaria

Miliaria (also called "sweat rash" or "prickly heat") is a skin disease marked by small and itchy rashes. Miliaria is a common ailment in hot and humid conditions such as in the tropics and during the summer season.

The level of obstruction within the eccrine duct determines the type of miliaria.

CLASSIFICATION

Type	Level of obstruction
Miliaria crystallina	Stratum corneum
Miliaria rubra	Stratum granulosum and below
Miliaria profunda	Dermoepidernal junction.

Common in a hot and humid environment.

MILIARIA RUBRA (PRICKLY HEAT)

Discrete, erythematous papules or papulovesicles often formed in sheets. Palms and soles are not affected. The eruption may sometimes be pruritic as well. Secondary bacterial infection.

Treatment: Air-conditioned surrounding or circulating air fans may provide considerable relief. Avoidance of exercise and tight or occlusive clothing is also helpful.

Systemic antibiotics indicated in the presence of secondary bacterial infection.

52. MILIUM

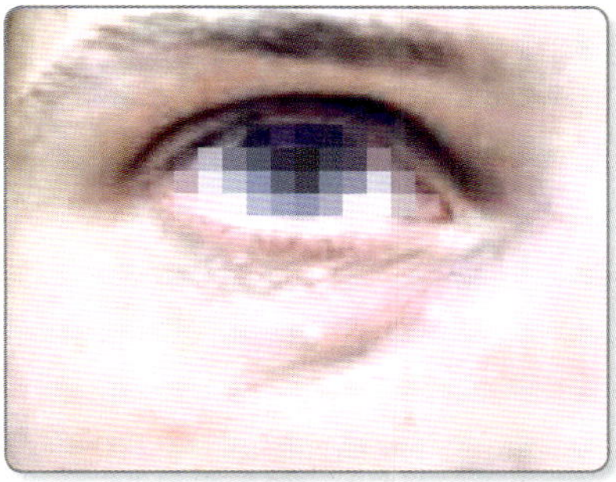

Milium

A tiny keratinous cyst following trauma to the skin. The latter can be in the form of burns, bulla formation as in epidermolysis bullosa and porphyrias, dermabrasion scars or radiodermatitis.

53. MOLLUSCUM CONTAGIOSUM

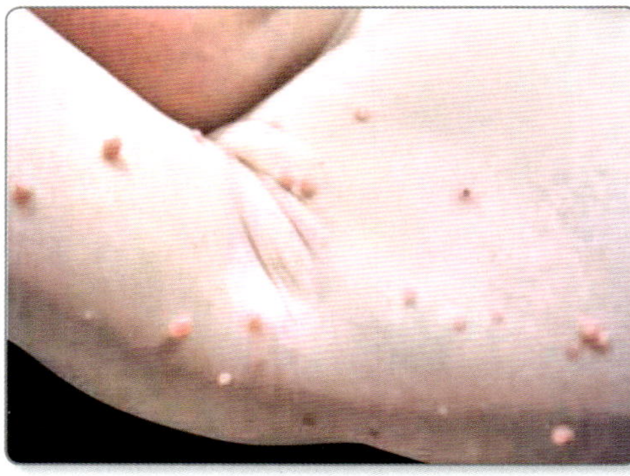

Molluscum contagiosum

Molluscum contagiosum (MC) is a viral infection of the skin or occasionally of the mucous membranes.

The virus commonly spreads through skin-to-skin contact.

Molluscum contagiosum lesions are flesh-colored, dome-shaped, and pearly in appearance. They are often 1–5 millimeters in diameter, with a dimpled center. They are generally not painful, but they may itch or become irritated.

It is an infectious disease caused by a pox virus molluscum contagiosum virus (MCV).

Many cells in the nodules contain ovoid intracytoplasmic eosinophilic inclusion bodies called "molluscum bodies."

The incubation period is 14–50 days. An individual lesion is shiny, pearly white, hemispherical umbilicated papules.

Treatment: Curettage after application of an anesthetic cream cryotherapy.

54. MONILIASIS (CANDIDIASIS)

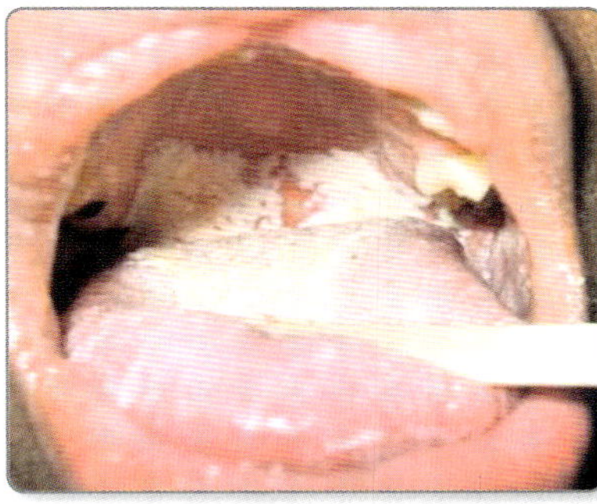

Moniliasis

Candidiasis is an infection caused by the yeast-like fungus *Candida albicans*. The infection is usually confined to the skin, nail, mucous membranes and gastrointestinal tract.

ETIOLOGY

In its yeast-like form, it is capable of producing long chain of elongated cells (pseudohyphae). The ability to exist in both hyphal and yeast forms is known as dimorphism.

CLINICAL DISEASE

Paronychia, endocarditis, otitis externa, vaginitis, intestinal, broncho-pulmonary, bone and joint, CNS and systemic infection, onchomyosis.

PREDISPOSING FACTORS

Trauma, moisture.
Nutritional factors: Avitaminosis, iron deficiency, generalized malnu-tririon, old age, pregnancy.
Systemic illnesses: Down's syndrome, acrodermatitis enteropathica, hypothyroidism, malignancy.

Immunodeficiency states, AIDS, corticosteroids and other immunosuppressive agents.

Treatment: Topical clotrimazole, miconazole, nystatin cream, amphotericin B, systemic therapy ketaconazole, itraconazole.

55. MORPHEA (LOCALIZED CIRCUMSCRIBED SCLERODERMA)

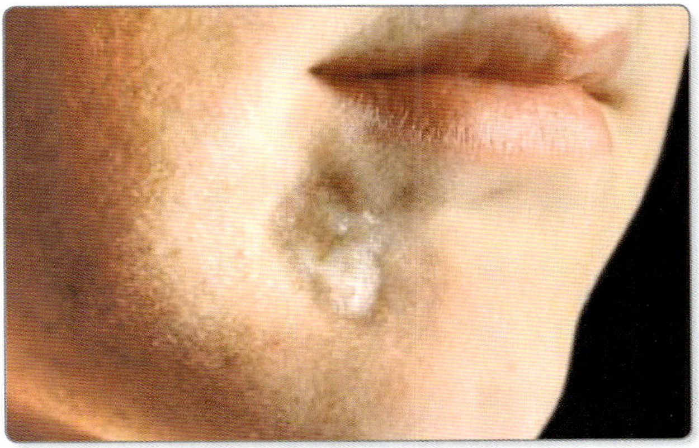

Morphea

It is a disorder of unknown cause wherein localized sclerosis of the skin occurs.

ETIOLOGY

The exact cause is unknown.

CLINICAL VARIANTS

1. Plaque type
2. Guttate lesions
3. Linear lesion
4. Segmental morphea
5. Subcutaneous morphea (Morphea profunda)

Treatment: Intralesional steroids, phenytoin sodium orally.

56. NEUROFIBROMA

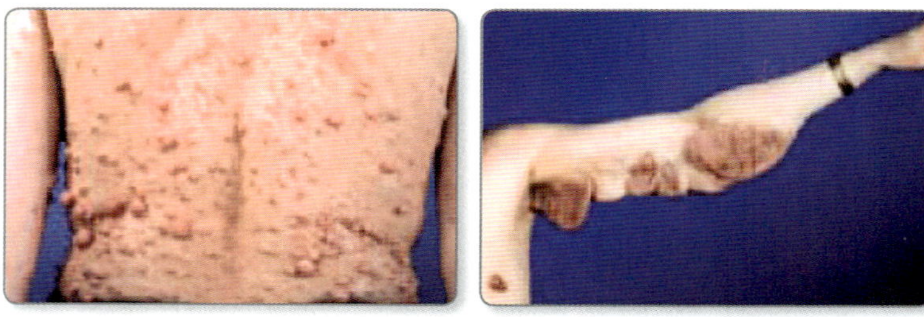

Neurofibroma

Autosomal dominant inheritance.

CLINICAL FEATURES

Soft tumors, sessiles and dome-shaped, sometimes pedunculated. Most numerous on the trunk and limbs. Cafe au lait spots, freckling, oral lesions, kyphoscoliosis, short stature and macrocephaly.
The pathogenesis is uncertain.

PATHOLOGY

Cutaneous neurofibromas are derived from peripheral nerves and their supporting structures.

Treatment: Symptomatic.

57. OIL FOLLICULITIS

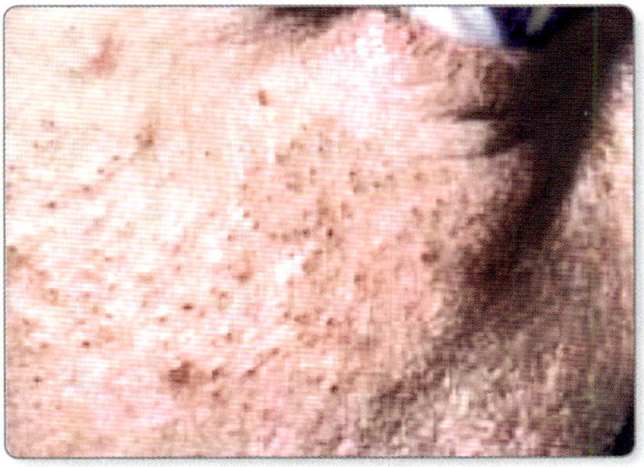

Oil folliculitis

One of the occupational dermatoses. Oil plugging of many follicles. Follicular papules, pinhead pustules. Pustules may be sterile or may contain coagulase negative Staphyloccocus.

Treatment: Remove contact with irritant oil. Use protective clothing, gloves, keratolytics.

58. PEDICULOSIS

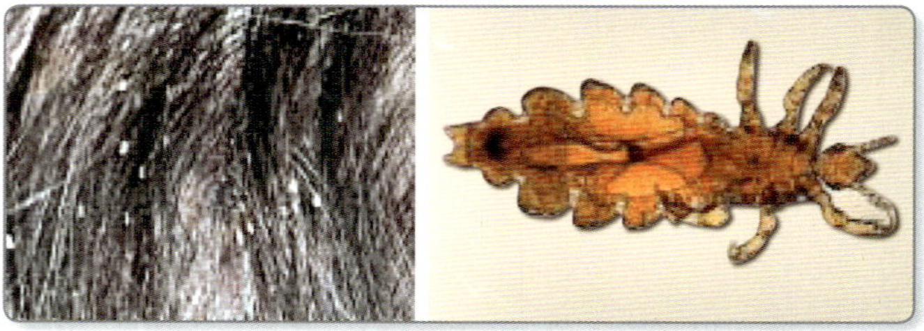

Pediculosis

Pediculosis is caused by sucking lice of the order Anoplura. There are three types of lice, *Pediculus humanus* var. *capitis*, the head louse; *Pediculus humanus* var. *corporis*, the body louse; and *Phthirus pubis*, the pubic louse. They are obligate parasites of man. The lice are six-legged insects.

Unless dislodged mechanically, lice spend their entire life on the host. They are transferred from one host to another by the slightest body contacts, or indirectly through the use of combs, brushes, caps, or clothings.

They take 2 to 3 blood meals per day. It is estimated that in a moderately severe infestation the lice suck about 10 to 20 ml of blood per day.

PEDICULOSIS CAPITIS

Overcrowding and poor hygiene, low socio-economic status favors this condition.

CLINICAL FEATURES

Pediculosis capitis remains localized to the scalp and rarely infest other hairy region of the body like the beard. The nits are overglistening, translucent, whitish capsule attached to the side of a hair by a firm chitinous sheath which encircles the hair shaft. Itching of the scalp is the predominent symptom.

Oozing, crusting and eczematization of the scalp with regional lymphadenopathy are common presentation. A generalized erythematous maculopapular rash mainly on the trunk can occur as a sensitization reaction to pediculosis, a pediculid.

Treatment: When there is secondary pyoderma, use of co-trimoxazole is essential. Topical use of DDT and gamma benzene hexachloride (Gammexane, lindane) permethrin.

PEDICULOSIS CORPORIS

The diagnosis is suspected by the parallel scratch marks and hyper-pigmentation, especially of the upper back. Diagnosis is confirmed by finding lice or nits in the clothing or in bedding.

PHTHIRUS PUBIS

Itching of the pubic region is usually the initial symptom. Later secondary infection and eczematization occur. Blue-gray macula cerulae, sometimes seen on the lower abdomen and are probably produced by altered blood pigment or a reaction to the louses saliva.

Treatment: Gammabenzene hexachloride as a lotion, cream or shampoo is effective therapy.

59. PEMPHIGUS

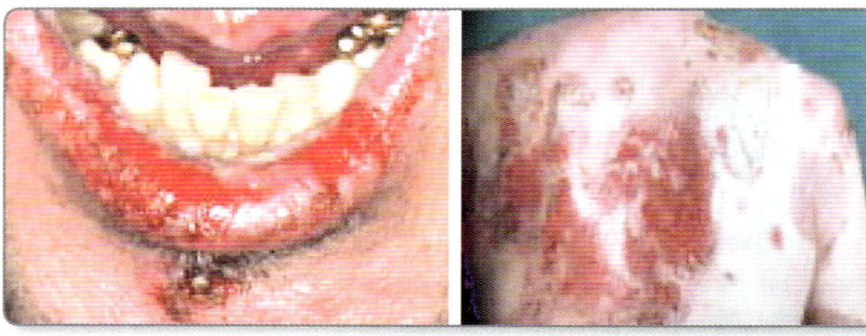

Pemphigus

"Pemphigus" is the collective term for a group of chronic bullous dermatoses characterized by an intraepidermal cleft and the presence of circulating autoantibodies directed against the cell surface of epithelial cells.

Diagnostic Features of Pemphigus Group of Diseases

	Clinical features	Histology
1. Pemphigus vulgaris	Oral lesions often precede flaccid bullae scalp, face axillae Nikolsky's sign positive	Suprabasal blister with acantholysis "Tombstone" appearance
2. Pemphigus vegetans	Bullae followed by hypertrophic. Pappillomatous lesions in intertriginous sites	Vegetating intraepidermal eosinophilic abscesses
3. Pemphigus foliaceus	Small flaccid bullae crust seborrheic areas; later generalized, Nikolsky's sign positive	Subcorneal or granular layer acantholytic blister. Dyskeratotic cells in granular layer
4. Pemphigus erythematosus	Erythematous scaly plaques and crusts on butterfly area of face, upper part of back chest and intertriginous areas	Mid epidermal cleavage. Similar to pemphigus foliaceus

Drug-induced pemphigus:

1. D-penicillamine
2. Sulfhydryl Group
3. Penicillin, ampicillin, amoxicillin, cefadroxil, rifampicin, propranolol, phenytoin and phenobarbitone.

Treatment: Corticosteroids, gold oral immunosuppressive drugs cyclophosphamide, cyclosporin azathioprine, methotrexate.

60. PHRYNODERMA

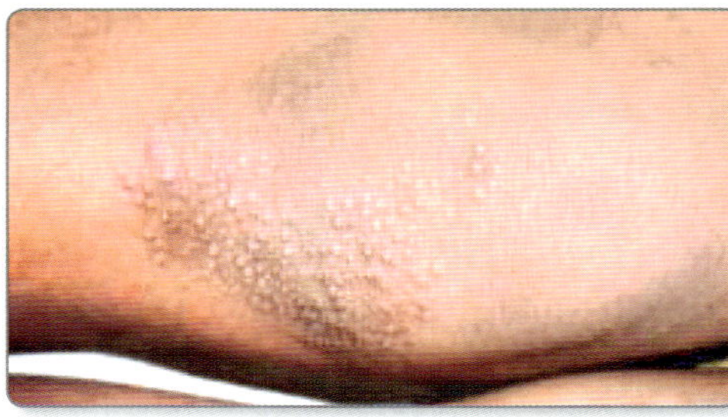

Phrynoderma

In hypovitaminosis A, follicular keratotic papules of various sizes are distributed over the extensor aspects of extremities especially over the elbows, knees and thighs. The present view is that phrynoderma is a manifestation not only of deficiency or vitamin A, but also of that of essential fatty acids, vitamin C and vitamin E. Various eye symptoms and signs such as night blindness, Bitot's spots, xerophthalmia and keratomalacia may be associated. Deficiency of other vitamins and essential fatty acid should also be corrected.

61. PITYRIASIS ALBA

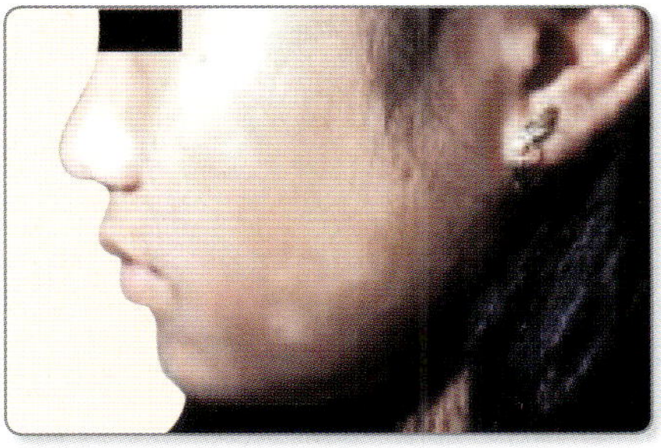

Pityriasis alba

Pityriasis alba is a common skin condition mostly occurring in children and usually seen as dry, fine-scaled, pale patches on the face. It is self-limiting and usually only requires use of moisturizer creams. This is a nonspecific dermatitis showing erythematous scaly patches usually over the face.

ETIOLOGY

Unknown. Precipitating causes are wind, soap and sunshine, atopy.

DIFFERENTIAL DIAGNOSIS

Pityriasis versicolor, early vitiligo and leprosy.

Treatment: Emollient, mild topical steroids.

62. PITYRIASIS ROSEA

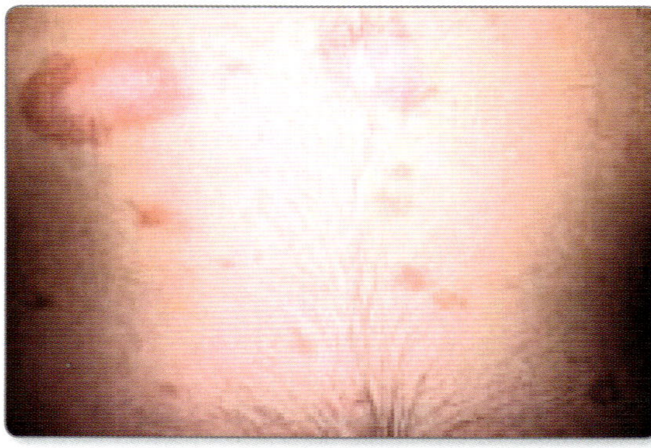

Pityriasis rosea

Pityriasis rosea is an acute self-limiting papulosquamous rash, probably infective in nature, mainly involving children and young adults. A primary lesion followed after an interval by a widespread. Virus-like particles have been detected ultrastructurally in some studies.

CLINICAL FEATURES

Constitutional symptoms like headache, malaise, arthralgia. The first manifestation is the herald patch or mother patch.

Erythematous, scaly, well-defined oval or round lesion. On the anterior aspect of the chest, back, neck, abdomen and extremities. The scales are fine and dry, from a collarette attached to the periphery.

Mucosal involvement can take different forms a single large erythematous platal plaque and scattered multiple tiny hemorrhagic puncta.

DIFFERENTIAL DIAGNOSIS

Drug rash, seborrheic dermatitis, secondary syphilis, ringworm.

Treatment: Symptomatic.

63. POROKERATOSIS (MIBELLI)

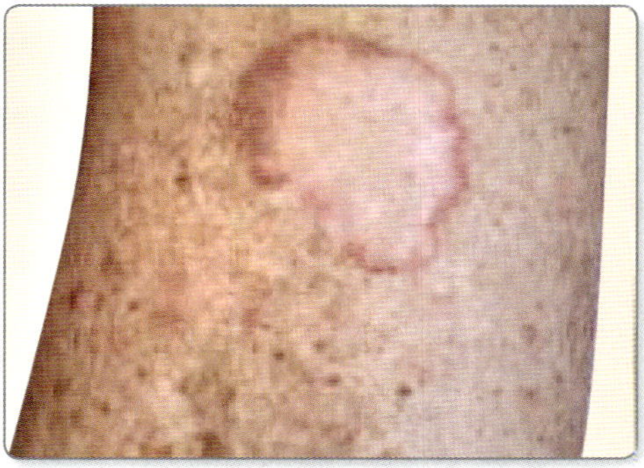

Porokeratosis

Porokeratosis or Mibelli is a genetic disease transmitted as an autosomal dominant trait. It is as common in males as in females.

CLINICAL FEATURES

As a tiny keratotic papule which slowly enlarges peripherally to form an annular seriginous plaque with central hyperpigmentation dryness and mild atrophy. Each lesion has characteristic peripheral slightly raised keratotic wall with a central groove. Mucosal lesions may occur. On the glands penis it may cause multiple erosions. When it occurs on the scalp cicatrical alopecia may result.

Different clinical types are the plaque, superficial disseminated. Superficial actinic, linear punctate and hypertropic or warty types. Malignant change can ocur in longstanding lesions of porokeratosis.

HISTOPATHOLOGY

Porokeratosis shows characteristic histopathological features. The ridge shows a keratin filled invagination of the epidermis. In the center of this invagination can be seen the most characteristic histologic feature, the cornoid lamella, a porokeratotic column.

64. PRURIGO

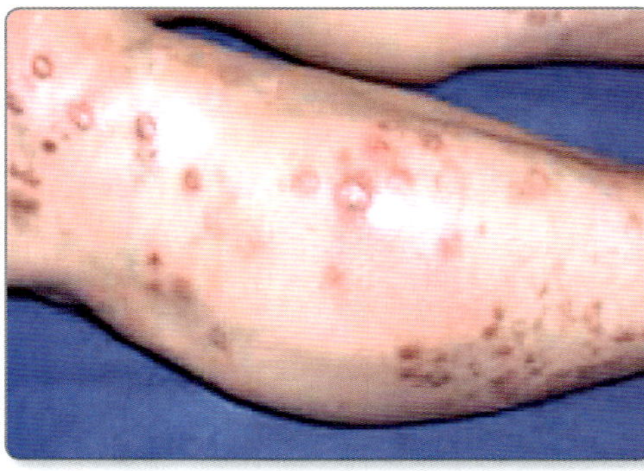

Prurigo

The term prurigo denotes a skin lesion usually a papule or nodule of unknown etiology, which is intensly pruritic.

Types: Simple acute prurigo is a synonym for papula urticaria. Subacute prurigo, chronic prurigo, dermographic prurigo, prurigo pigmentosa, prurigo nodularis.

65. PRURITUS

Itching or pruritus often can be defined as a cutaneous sensation that produces the desire to scratch.

DERMATOLOGICAL CONDITIONS

1. Atopic eczema
2. Xerosis
3. Scabies of the clean
4. Ectoparasitic infestation
5. Urticaria
6. Lichen planus
7. Dermatitis herpetiformis.

SYSTEMIC CAUSE OF PRURITUS

I. Endocrine and Metabolic
1. Diabetes mellitus
2. Gout
3. Hyper- and hypo-thyroidism
4. Hyper- and hypo-parathyroidism.

II. Hepatic
1. Pregnancy pruritus

III. Renal
Chronic renal failure

IV. Hematopoietic Disease
1. Polycythemia rubra vera
2. Iron deficiency
3. Mastocytosis.

V. Malignancies

VI. Allergy
1. Intestinal parasites
2. Food

VII. Drug

VIII. Neurological

IX. Psychoneurosis

LABORATORY TESTS

1. Hematologic
   - Complete blood count
   - Serum iron
   - Serum protein electrophoresis
   - Erythrocyte sedimentation rate (ESR)
2. Hepatic
   - Serum glutamic oxaloacetic transaminase (SGOT)
   - Bilirubin
   - Alkaline phosphatase
3. Renal
   - Blood urea nitrogen (BUN) and creatinine
   - Urine analysis
4. Endocrine
   - Thyroid
   - Glucose tolerance test (GTT)
   - Chest X-ray
5. Stool examination for parasites and occult blood

Treatment: Elimination of provocative factors, topical therapy calamine lotion, systemic therapy, antihistamines.

66. PSORIASIS

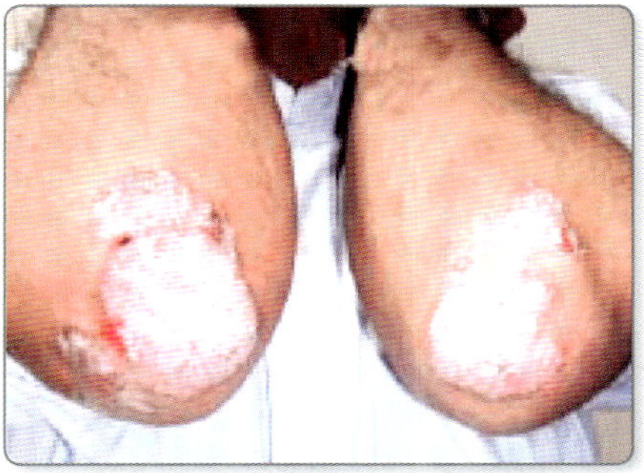

Psoriasis

Psoriasis is defined as chronic inflammatory disease of the skin of unknown cause characterized by erythematous papules or plaques covered with dry silvery scales with or without arthropathy. Any age can be affected. Both sexes are equally affected. Auspitz's sign is positive. Koebner phenomenon is often present.

GENETIC FACTORS

HLA-B13, HLA-B17 and HLA-Bw16 in patient with psoriasis.

HISTOPATHOLOGICAL FACTORS

Porokeratosis, uniform, presence of 'microabscesses of Munro' in the horny layers, absence of granular layers, regular elongation of rete ridges, regular elongation of the dermal papillae, which are clubbed at their upper portions. There are dilated and tortuous capillaries in the papillae with edema and perivascular mononuclear cells infiltration. There is thinning of the suprapapillary parts of the stratum malpighii with the occasional presence of a small spongiform pustules.

TRIGGERING FACTORS

Trauma may be of any kind physical, chemical, mechanical, allergic. Seasonal variations. Pregnancy, remission of psoriasis may occur during pregnancy but there is exacerbation during the postpartum period. Emotional stress. Psoriasis is more stress sensitive infection, upper respiratory tract infections tonsilitis especially when caused by streptococcal may cause a flare-up of existing psoriasis. Drugs: beta blocking drugs, lithium.

DIFFERENTIAL DIAGNOSIS

Seborrheic dermatitis, pityriasis rosea, lichen planus, syphilis secondary stage, Tinea (Fungus), drug reactions.
Clinical classification of psoriasis:

1. Guttate psoriasis
2. Chronic plaque psoriasis
3. Exfoliative psoriasis
4. Pustular psoriasis
5. Psoriasis unguals
6. Arthropathic psoriasis
7. Regional variations in psoriasis; scalp face, flexural psoriasis, scrotum, napkin area, palms and soles
8. Nail-pitting

Treatment: General measures: Treat the provocating factors. Topical salicyclic acid, tar, anthralin (Dithranol), calcipotriol corticosteroids. Systemic drugs: Oral retinoids, methotrexate, psoralens (PUNA therapy), immunosuppressive drugs.

67. REITER'S DISEASE

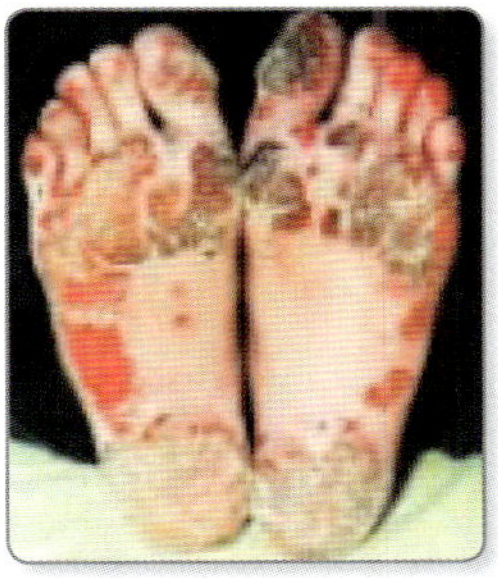

Reiter's disease

The cause is unknown. The most constant features are polyarthritis and nongonococcal urethritis with conjunctivitis or iritis. It may be seen in association with venerally acquired urethritis or as a complication of dysentery or nonspecific diarrhea.

The characteristics lesion of the skin is keratoderma blennorrhagica.

Treatment: Tetracycline, analgesic, corticosteroids.

68. ROSACEA

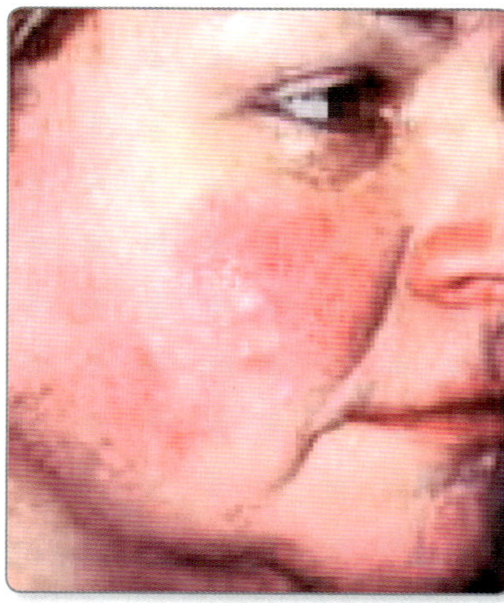

Rosacea

Rosacea is generally grouped with acne vulgaris because of a similar involvement of the face, the appearance of papular pustular lesions, and its response to tetracycline.

Affects the flush area of the face, manifestating with telangiectasis, erythema and papulopustular lesion; chronic course.
Rhinophyma is a complication.

CLINICAL FEATURES

Exacerbations occur with emotional stress, excess alcohol, heat, sun exposure, vasodilators and hot food. Occular rosacea is seen. Involvement of the eyes with blepharitis, conjunctivitis, episcleritis, keratitis and iritis.

Treatment: Patients should avoid exposure to whatever that make their skin flush. Tetracycline.

69. SCABIES

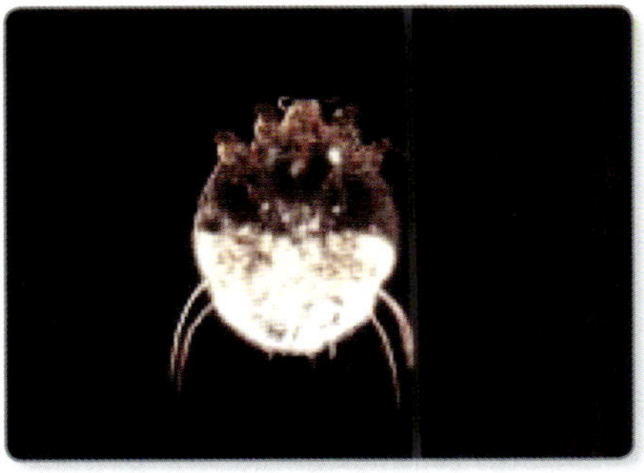

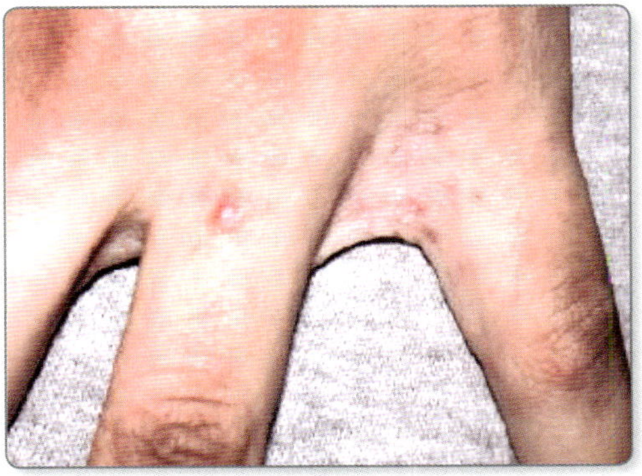

Scabies

EPIDEMIOLOGY

Scabies is contracted by direct intimate contact with an infected person. Overcrowding and poor hygiene facilitates the infection and indirect spread by clothing and bedding.

Scabies is a highly contagious, pruritic disease caused by itch mite. Sarcoptes scabiei var homins. Sarcoptes scabiei are hemispherical mites, is about 0.4/0.3 mm. They have four pairs of leg. In female, the front two pairs end in the suckers.

The male is much smaller (0.2/0/15) and his fourth pair of legs also end in suckers. Only the fertilized female can burrow into the skin. She extends her burrow by about 2 mm and deposits 2 to 3 eggs per day. She lays about 10 to 30 eggs.

The six, legged larvae emerge from the eggs after 3 or 4 days, wander to the skin surface and form shallow pockets in the original or a new host. Copulation occurs in the pocket and the female excavates her burrow, whilst the male soon dies. Hands and wrists, the elbow, feet, axilla, thigh, penis and scrotum are the sites affected.

Face, palm and sole also in infancy but not in adult.

CLINICAL FEATURES

Itching is the predominant symptom. Nocturnal worsening of itching is highly characteristic. Scabies involves the webs of the fingers flexor aspects of the wrist, elbow anterior axillary fold, umbilicus and periumbilical region, the genitalia and upper thighs, knees and ankles. In the female, the nipple and areola are also involved. The lower parts of the buttocks and natal left are common sites.

The burrow is the pathognominic lesion of scabies. It is a serpentine, thread like, grayish or dark line. Small erythematous papules or papulovesicles. Lesion are often excoriated and secondarily infected.

1. Scabies in babies. 2. Scabies in healthy and clean adults. 3. Crusted scabies (Norwegian). 4. Scabies incognito. 5. Animal transmitted scabies. 6. Nodular scabies.

COMPLICATION

Secondary pyoderma as impetigo, ecythyma and furunculosis are most common complications. Acute glomerulonephritis is the systematic complication.

Treatment: The medicine is preferably applied after a good scrub with soap and water.

All the clothes he has worn during the period of treatment should be washed and dried in the hot sun or ironed. All members of the personal household and other intimate contract should be treated even if they do not have obvious symptoms or sign. One percent Gamma benzene hexachloride, permethrin, 25% benzyl benzoate, crotamiton, malathion (0.5% liquid). Treatment of complication important 10–15% sulfur ointment can be used.

70. SCROFULODERMA

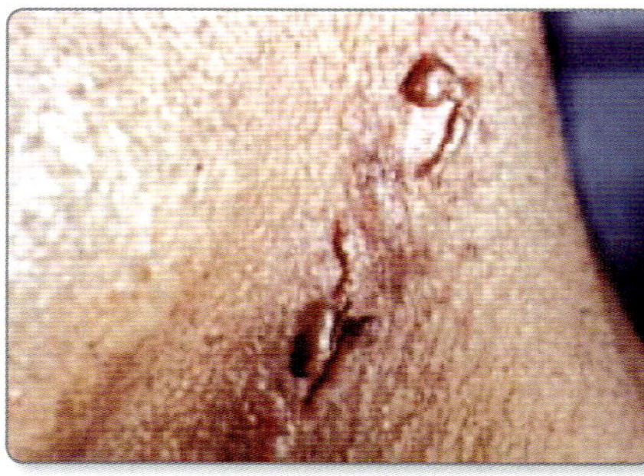

Scrofuloderma

It is a type of cutaneous tuberculosis. Breakdown of the skin overlying a tuberculous, focus, usually a lymph gland or joint or bone. Caseation necrosis usually seen in the deeper dermis.

Treatment: Anti-tuberculosis drugs.

71. SEBORRHEIC DERMATITIS
(SYN. DERMATITIS OF THE SEBACEOUS AREA)

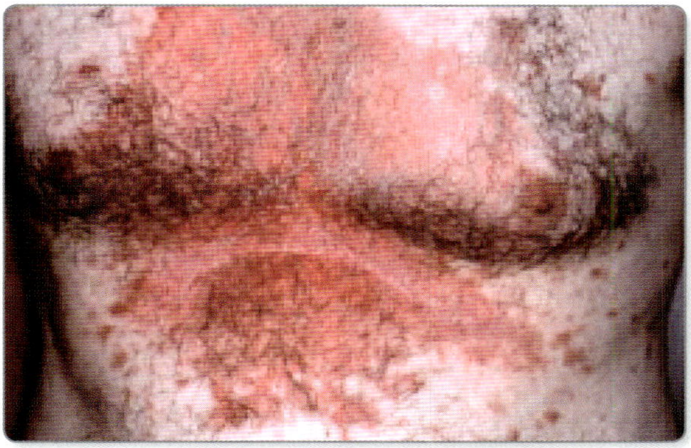

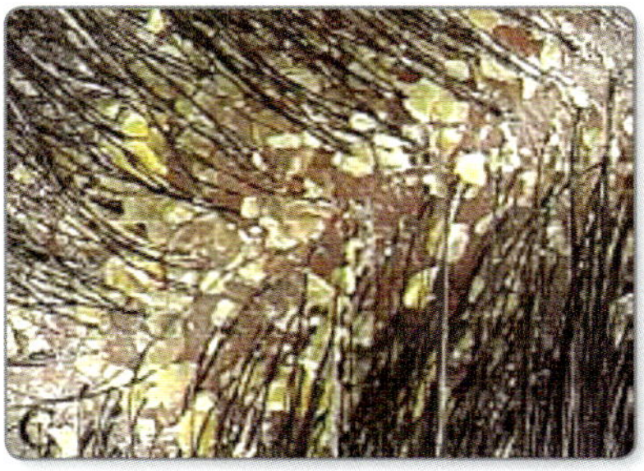

Seborrheic dermatitis

The term seborrhea denotes increased secretion of the sebaceous glands resulting in excessive oiliness of the skin. The yeast *Pityrosporum ovale* is probably causative factor, but both genetic and environmental factors influence the onset of disease.

CLINICAL FEATURES

Infants

The first few days or weeks of life, commonly between the third and eighth weeks as greasy scaling in the scalp, they are so-called cradle cap. Small, round or oval, erythematous scaly lesions are seen on the face and the napkin area.

The prognosis even without any treatment is good.

Adults

Seborrheic dermatitis is more common in winter than in summer. Lesion may be present on the hairy skin of the scalp, face and behind the ears, preretinal and interscapular region, flexures (inflammatory folds, axillae, groins, anogenital folds) and around the umbilicus.

Scalp Dandruff denotes an exaggerated loss of keratinized cells from the surface of the scalp.

Face Areas of the erythema and scaling involve the nasolabial folds.

Trunk Seborrheic dermatitis has been recently found to be associated with AIDS and the AIDS related complex.

Treatment: Topical application of selenium sulfide, low potency steroid cream; more severe cases—sulfur and salicyclic acid preparation.

72. SUN AND SKIN PHOTOSENSITIVE DERMATOSES

This is caused or precipitated or aggravated by sunlight.

	Classification Disease
1. Photoaggravated dermatoses	Lupus erythematosus, dermatomyositis, Darier's disease, lichen planus actinicus, pemphigus foliaceus
2. Genetic and metabolic dermatoses	Xeroderma pigmentosum, porphyria, pellagra, Hartnup's disease
3. Degenerative and neoplastic	Actinic keratoses squamous cell carcinoma, basal cell carcinoma, malignant melanoma
4. Phototoxic dermatoses	Contactants drugs/chemicals
5. Photoallergic dermatoses	Contactants drugs/chemicals
6. Idiopathic photodermatoses	Polymorphic light eruption Hydroa vacciniforme actinic Prurigo solar urticaria chronic Actinic dermatitis Actinic reticuloid

73. SYCOSIS BARBAE

Chronic infection (pyogenic) involving whole depth of hair follicle, beard male. Discrete red follicular pustules. Follicle surrounded by chronic granulomatous infiltrate lymphocytes, plasma cells, and histiocytes.

Treatment: Antibiotics.

74. SYPHILIS

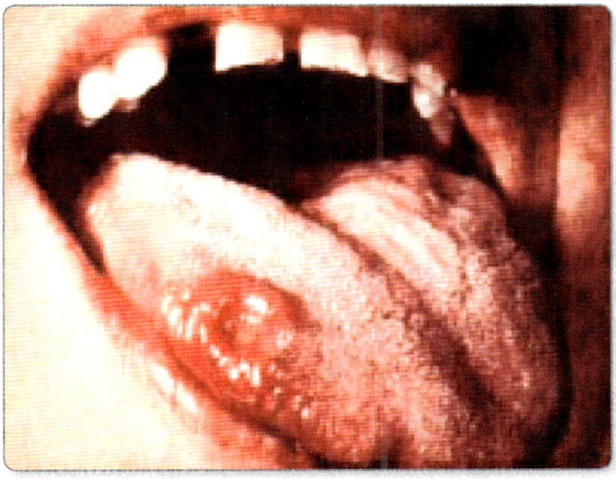

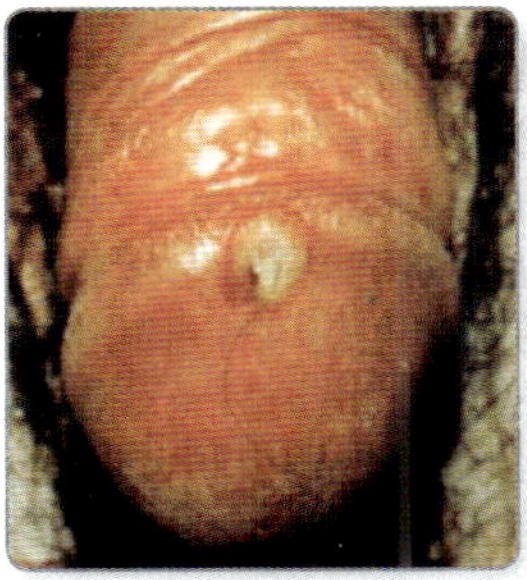

Syphilis

Causative organism *Treponema pallidum*. It is a delicate thread-like spiral parasite.

TRANSMISSION

In acquired syphilis this may be direct infection through sexual intercourse. Congenital syphilis is transmitted by an infected mother, usually in the early stages of the disease, by transplacental passage of the organism into the bloodstream of the fetus.

PATHOLOGY

The essential lesion in all phases of the syphilis is the same being strikingly characterized by perivascular round cell infiltration mainly lymphocyte and to a lesser extent by plasma and mononuclear cells.

CLINICAL FEATURES

Primary stage occurs between 10 and 28 days after infection. The primary lesion or chancre is an indurated, inflammatory, papular lesion usually ulcerated and covered with exudate. The site most commonly affected is the corona sulcus, but any area of the penis. The regional adenitis is common and malaise is often present.

SECONDARY STAGE

This occurs between 6 weeks and 2 years after the appearance of the chancre, and lasts about 2 years. Patients show skin lesion, generalized lymphadenopathy oral and tonsillar lesion, and a very small number have involvement of the nervous system, bones, eyes and abdominal viscera.

CLINICAL FEATURES

Lesions first to appear are macular, or maculopapular, early lesion, macular, maculopapular, papular, late lesion, annular, pustular, psoriasiform.

Other Signs

Alopecia, jaundice may occur in severe infection, secondary anemia, generalized lymphadenopathy, atrophy of the skin.

TERTIARY STAGE

Lesions are all gummatous. Types of gummata:

1. Nodular
2. Squamous

Other Signs

Bursitis of elbow joint, acromial process of the scapula, and extensortendons of the fingers. Cardiovascular, CNS and visceral complications.

Treatment: Early syphilis (Primary, secondary, less than 1 year)

1. Benzathine penicillin 2.4 mega units 1 mg
2. Tetracycline 500 mg 1Q1D × 15 days
3. Erythrocin 500 mg 1Q1D × 15 days.

   Late syphilis: Benzathine penicillin 2.4 million units per week for 3 doses (Total 7.2 million units)

   Tetracycline 500 mg 1Q1D × 30 days

   Erythrocin 500 mg 1Q1D × 30 days

75. SYSTEMIC SCLERODERMA

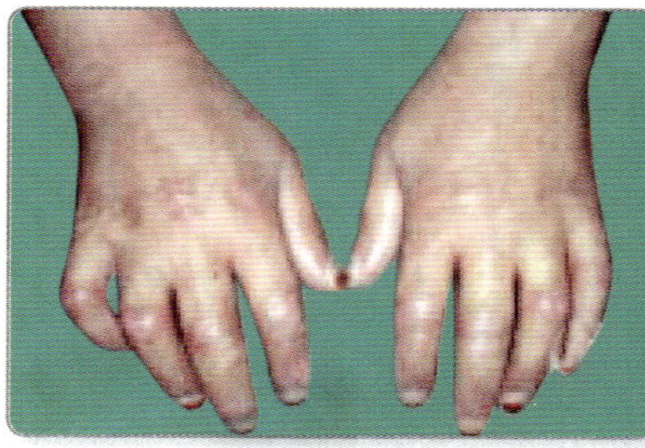

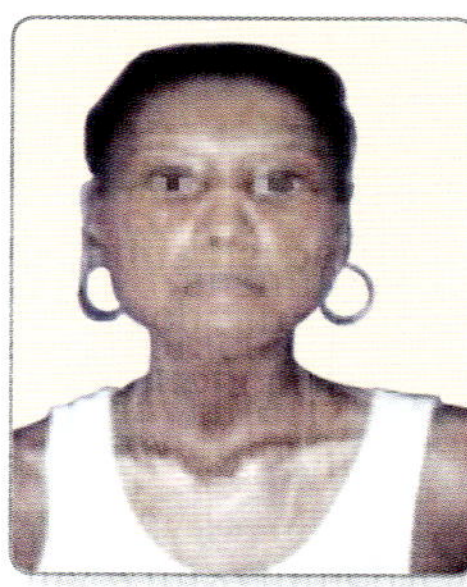

Scleroderma

Systemic scleroderma is a progressive often fatal, disorder characterized by the diffuse involvement of the connective tissue of the dermis leading to induration and thickening of the skin and fibrous deposition in certain internal organs. The other type is limited cutaneous scleroderma or acrosclerosis. A further variant known as the CREST occurs over extremities and face.

CUTANEOUS CHANGES

1. Sclerodactyly
2. Bibasilar pulmonary fibrosis
3. Pigmentation
4. Calcinosis
5. Gangrene and leg ulcers

INVOLVEMENT OF INTERNAL ORGANS

- Gastrointestinal involvement
- Hepatic involvement
- Pulmonary involvement
- Cardiac involvement
- Renal involvement
- Muscle involvement
- Bone changes
- Nervous system involvement
- Ocular involvement

Treatment: Corticosteroids, physiotherapy and penicillamine.

76. TINEA VERSICOLOR

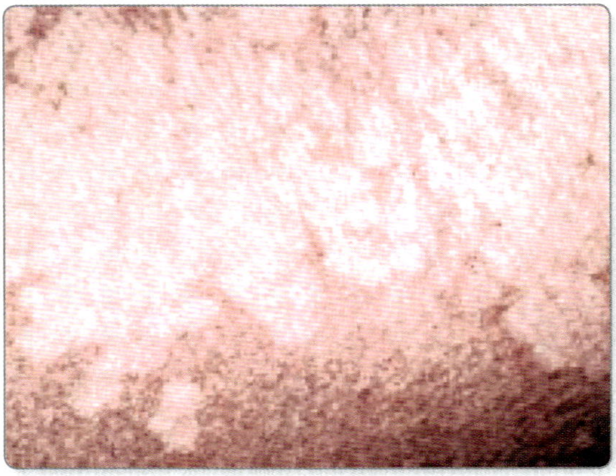

Tinea versicolor

Opportunistic infection by *Pityrosporum orbiculare* (Syn, *Malassezia furfur*) affect mainly stratum corneum in the form of scaly hypo-and hyper-pigmented macules.

DIFFERENTIAL DIAGNOSIS

Pityriasis alba, pityriasis rosea, vitiligo, secondary syphilis, leprosy seborrheic eczema.

Treatment: Selenium sulfide suspension, 2.5% sodium hyposulfate, salicylic acid ointment, imidazole group, ketoconazole.

77. TRICHOMONIASIS

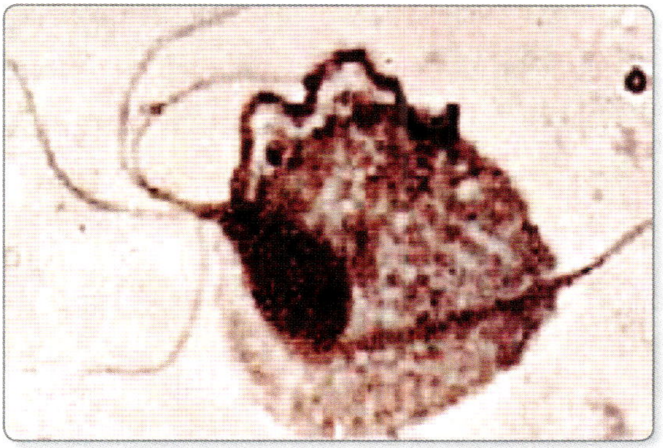

Trichomoniasis

A common sexually transmitted disease (STD). Both men and women are affected. Caused by a protozoan *Trichomonas vaginalis*. Vaginal infections in women and urethral infections in men. Genital itching and/or burning, vaginal or vulval redness, frothy yellow-green vaginal discharge with a strong odor, frequent and/or painful urination, discomfort during intercourse and abdominal pain. Men are usually asymptomatic, but if a man has symptoms, they can include: Unusual penile discharge, painful urination, burning sensation after ejaculation, tingling inside the penis. Treatment: Antibiotics–Metronidazole 500 mg 2–3 times a day for 7–10 days.

78. TUBERCULIDES

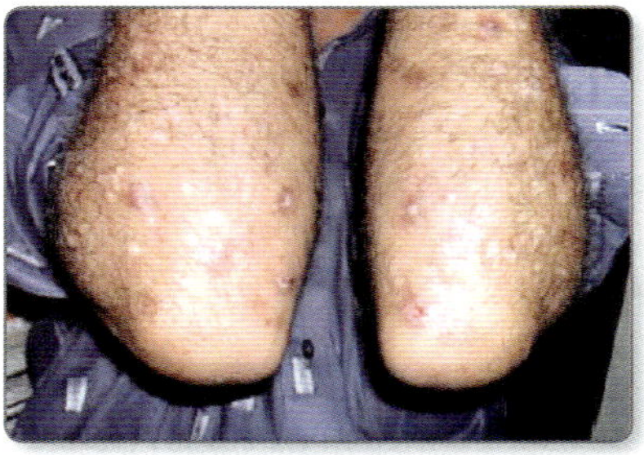

Tuberculides

A group of eruption which arise in response to an internal focus of tuberculosis and clear with anti-tuberculosis therapy.

Types: Papular and nodular tuberculides.

Papular type: Papulonecrotic, lichen scrofulosorum, Acne scrofulosorum and lichenoid tuberculides.

Nodular tuberculides: Erythema nodusum, erythema induratum, nodular vasculitis.

79. TUBERCULOSIS VERRUCOSA CUTIS (TBVC)

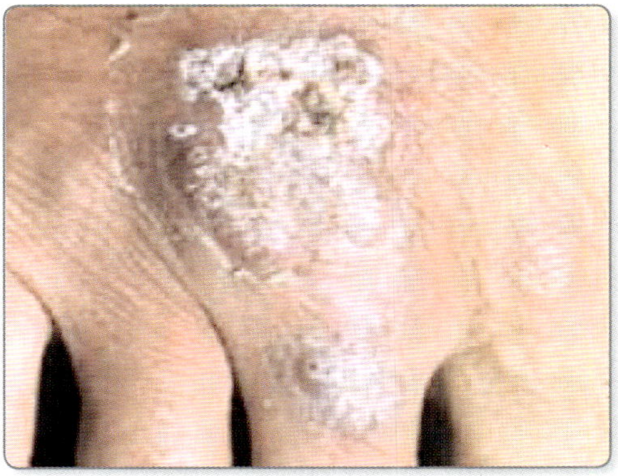

Tuberculosis verrucosa cutis

It is an occupational hazard in persons who handle tuberculosis tissues during their work, e.g. veterinarians. A dull red deeply seated papule or nodule gradually enlarge and becomes verrucous. Because of good immunity, the regional lymph nodes are not often enlarged.

On histology, pseudoepitheliomatous hyperplasia inflammatory infiltrate and rarely bacilli.

The disease should be differentiated from common was, plastomycosis, hypertrophic lichen planus and oriental sore in an endemic areas.

Treatment: Antituberculous drugs, streptomycin, INH, PAS, rifampicin.

80. TYLOSIS

Hyperkeratosis of palm, sole may be genetic or acquired. The commonest genetic type is Thost-Unna syndrome. Commonest of hereditary palmoplantar keratoderma. Predispose to esophageal carcinoma.

81. URTICARIA

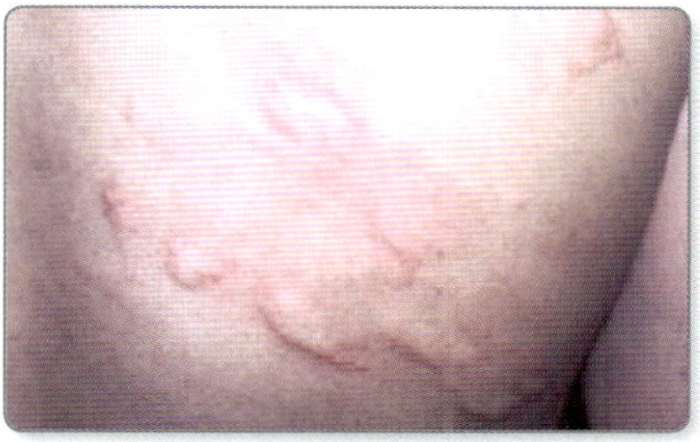

Urticaria

Urticaria consists of raised erythematous wheals which are pruritic.

PATHOLOGY

The mast cells are degranulated in urticaria.

PROVOKING CAUSES

Drug, food, parasites, inhalant, cholinergic, pressure and idiopathic, septic facus, cold, drug inhalants, infection and infestation, food additives, emotional stress, medical disease.

Treatment: Identify the provoking factors and treat accordingly, systemic antihistamine and corticosteroids.

82. VITILIGO

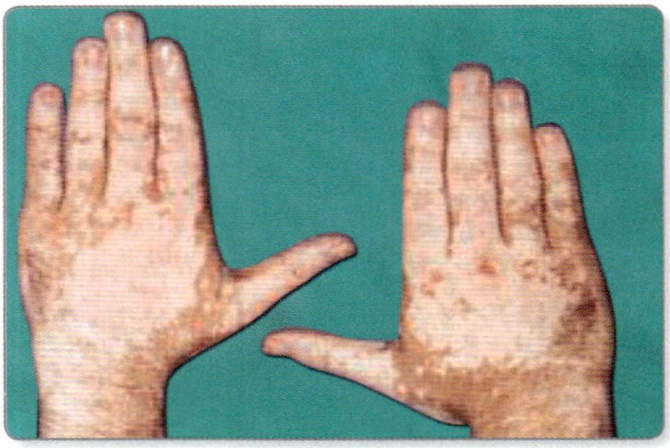

Vitiligo

Obscure etiology, clinically manifested by circumscribed achromic macules histologically by degeneration and disappearance of melanocyte in the involved skin.

ETIOPATHOGENESIS

Immune hypothesis, neural hypothesis, autotoxic, self-destructive or free radical hypothesis.

ASSOCIATED SYSTEMIC DISORDERS

Such disorders included pernicious anemia. Addison's disease, Grave's diseases, hyperthyroidism, hypothyroidism, thyroiditis hyperparathyroidism, diabetes mellitus, rheumatic disorders and internal malignancy.

83. WARTS (VERRUCAE)

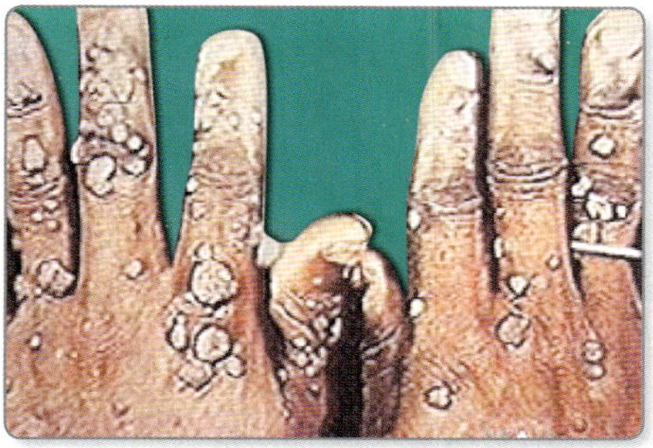

Warts

Cutaneous growth caused by human papilloma virus. They are contagious and autoinoculable. They are acquired by direct and indirect contact with contaminated objects.

All ages and both sexes are affected.

VARIOUS MORPHOLOGICAL TYPES OF WARTS

- Common warts or verruca vulgaris
- Plane wart or verruca plana
- Filiform and digitate warts
- Plantar warts
- Genital HPV infection - Condyloma accuminatum.

Treatment

- Suggestion therapy or hypnosis.
- Keratolytic agents
- Cytotoxic such as podophyllin, 20% podophyllin in Tr. benzoin co 5-fluorouracil
- Trichloroacetic acid 35%
- Formalin 10%
- Cryotherapy
- Curettage
- Interferon
- Electrodesiccation
- Excision
- Carbon dioxide laser

84. XANTHOMA

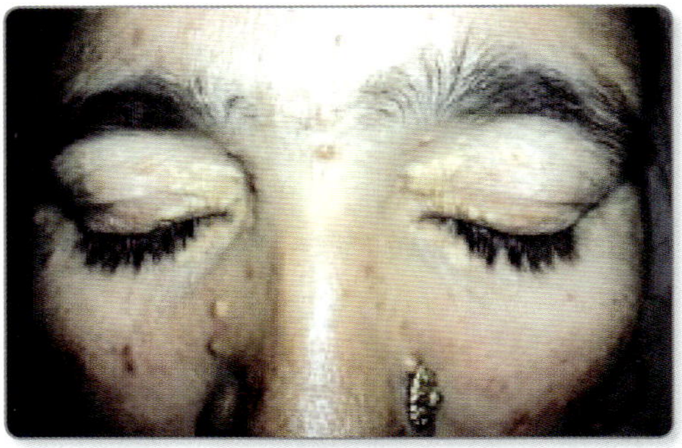

Xanthoma

A xanthoma is an uncommon presentation of a localized disturbance of lipid metabolism. An increased risk of arteriosclerotic vascular disease is present.

TYPES

Palpebral xanthoma, tuberous xanthoma, nodular xanthomas, generalized plane xanthoma disseminatum.

ERUPTIVE XANTHOMAS

They may occur suddenly over the buttocks, flexors of the arm, shoulders, thighs, knees, inguinal and axillary folds.

Treatment: Most of these respond to dietary control and drug therapy.

85. XERODERMA PIGMENTOSUM

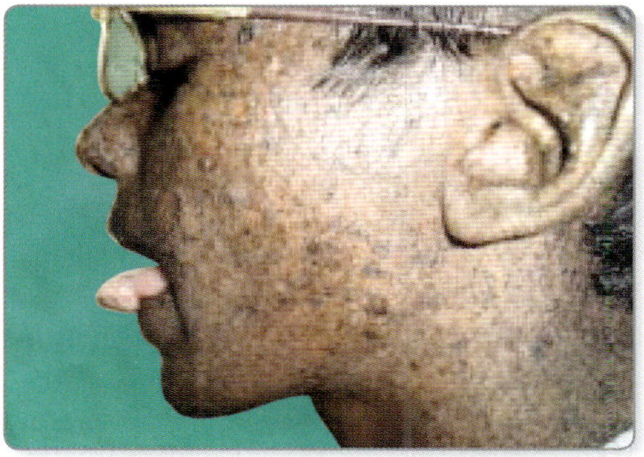

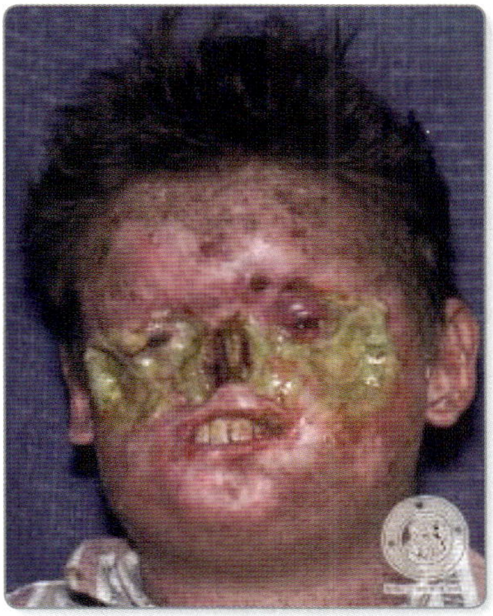

Xeroderma pigmentosum

An autosomal recessive disease associated with defective DNA repair. It is characterized by severe sun sensitivity resulting in progressive degenerative changes of the skin and eyes, leading to neoplasia early in life.

Both sexes are affected.

Etiopathogenesis

The gene responsible for this disorder may be located on chromosome 9 or 2. Normal (DNA repair proficient) cells are able to tolerate higher doses of UV - radiation and certain chemical carcinogens than XP cells.The DNA excision repair in human cell is defective in 80% of cases.

CLINICAL FEATURE

The first is characterized by photosensitivity between six months and three years of age. Erythema or blister appears on exposed areas.

Conjunctivitis and photophobia. The pigmentation stage usually begins by the age of two years as freckle.

The telangiectatic and atrophic stage is the combination of hypo- and hyper-pigmented macules, atrophy and telangiectasia is called poikiloderma. Benign growth, actinic keratosis and keratoacanthoma appear in the exposed areas in the next stage. Malignant tumors develop in almost all patients early in life.

NEUROLOGICAL FEATURES

Mental retardation, spasticity, deafness and EEG abnormalities.

PROGNOSIS

Most patient with the full-blown syndrome die within the first two decade.

Treatment: Early diagnosis, life long protection from UV exposure and early detection of neoplasms are essential. Strict photoprotection, surgery or chemotherapy of tumors and care of eyes are the mainstays of treatment.

86. ZOON'S PLASMA CELL BALANITIS

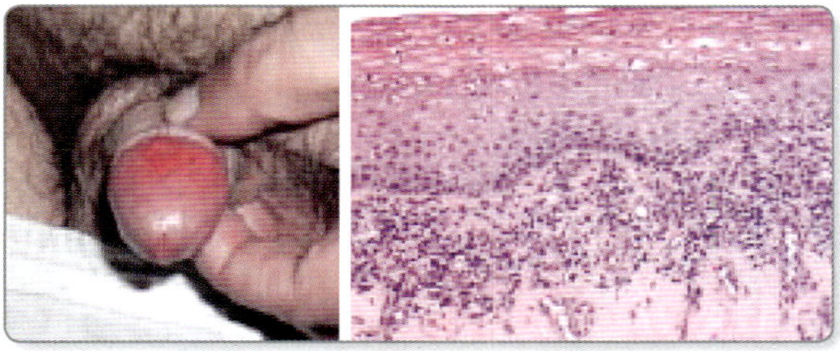

Zoon's plasma cell balanitis

1. Middle aged men.
2. Persistent chronic balanitis glans penis and prepuce.
3. Cayenne pepper spots over the surface is very characteristic.

Treatment: Topical steroids and circumcision.

HISTOPATHOLOGY OF FEW IMPORTANT CONDITIONS OF PEMPHIGUS

Select early vesicle for biopsy. Loss of coherence between epidermal cells (Acantholysis). The bulla in the suprabasal zone. The basal cells remain attached to the dermis producing a tombstone appearance. Acantholytic cells are present in the bulla cavity. These are rounded cells with loss of intracellular bridges, and peripheral condensation of the cytoplasm. There is scanty perivascular inflammatory infiltrate composed of lymphocytes, histocytes and occasional eosinophils and neutrophils and plasma cells.

LICHEN PLANUS

There is hyperkeratosis, focal hypergranulosis, irregular acanthosis damage to basal cell layer and a “band like” dermal infiltrate hugging the epidermis. The rete ridges show irregular lengthening giving them a saw-toothed appearance. The basal cell show liquefaction degeneration. There is incontinence of pigment which is taken up by melanophages in the upper dermis. Colloid, hyaline, or civatte bodies are seen.

LICHEN NITIDUS

The characteristic infiltrate is just below flattened epidermis and is well circumscribed. It consists of lymphocytes, histiocytes and a few Langhans giant cells and plasma cells. The adjacent epidermis extends around the infiltrate in a claw-like manner. There is liquefaction degeneration of the basal layer.

MOLLUSCUM CONTAGIOSUM

Cellular proliferation of the lower layers of the stratum malpighii produces multiple closely packed, pear-shapped lobules which compress the papillae. They appear as fibrous septa between the lobules. Many cells in the lobules contain ovoid intracytoplasmic eosinophilic inclusion bodies are called molluscum bodies.

MORPHEA

The epidermis may be normal or flattened and atrophic with loss of rete ridges. The dermis appears edematous with swelling, degeneration of collagen fibrils. The collagen becomes homogenous and eosinophilic. A slight perivascular lymphocytic infiltrate may be present. In the later stages the dermis is markedly thickened with dense collagen. The dermal appendages and subcutaneous fat are progressively lost.

PSORIASIS

1. Porokeratosis uniform
2. Microabscesses of Munro in the horny layer neutrophils. The spongiform pustules 3. Absence of granular layer 4. Regular elongation of a rete ridges 5. Regular elongation of the dermal papillae which are clubbed at their upper portions. They are dilated and tortuous capillaries in the papillae 6. Thinning of the suprapapillary parts of the stratum malpighii occasional presence of spongiform pustules.

WARTS

Hyperplasia of all layers of the epidermis with acanthosis, papillomatosis and hyperkeratotic porokeratosis. The rete ridges are elongated and in the periphery of the lesion are often bent inward. A characteristic feature is the presence of large vacuolated cells with round deeply basophilic nuclei. The nuclei of both types of cells contain numerous viral particles.

GLOSSARY OF CLINICAL AND HISTOPATHOLOGICAL TERMS

ABSCESS

It is a localized accumulation of purulent material, deep in the dermis and subcutaneous tissue.

ACANTHOLYSIS

This refers to the loss of cohesion between neighboring epidermal cells subsequent to the damage in the region of desmosome, e.g. pemphigus vulgaris, pemphigus foliaceus, benign familial pemphigus, and Darier's disease.

CRUST

It develops when serum, blood and purulent exudate dries on the skin surface.

CYST

It is a sac that contains fluid or semisolid material.

DYSKERATOSIS

It denotes premature or abnormal keratinization of individual epidermal cells.

EROSION

An erosion is a well-circumscribed loss of superficial layers epidermis.

FURUNCLES

A furuncle is a deep necrotizing form of folliculitis with pus accumulation.

GRANULOMA

Granuloma is an expression of delayed hypersensitivity reaction. It is characterized by collection of mononuclear cells in association with either epitheloid cells and/or multinucleated giant cells. Tuberculosis, leprosy, sarcoidosis, and deep mycoses are chronic granulomatous disorders.

HYPERKERATOSIS

It denotes an increase in the thickness of stratum corneum.

LICHENIFICATION

It is a reaction pattern to repeated rubbing which results in proliferation of the keratinocytes and stratum corneum.

MACULE

It is a well-circumscribed change in the color of the skin flushed to the skin surface.

NODULE

It is a palpable, solid, round or ellipsoidal lesion. Nodules may be located in the epidermis or may extend into the dermis and subcutaneous tissue.

PAPULE

It is a well-circumscribed solid elevated lesion less than 5 mm or 1 mm in diameter.

PLAQUE

It is a well-circumscribed alteration in the consistency/texture of the skin that may be either raised or depressed below the surface of the surrounding skin. Plaques are often by coalescence of papules.

POROKERATOSIS

In complete keratinization characterized by retention of the nuclei in the stratum corneum.

PSEUDOEPITHELIOMATOUS HYPERPLASIA

It is a reaction pattern of the skin to widely varying etiology characterized by irregular growth pattern of the acanthotic epidermis that has a tendency to invade the dermis.

PUSTULE

It is a well-circumscribed lesion that contain purulent exudate containing leukocytes.

SCALING

Abnormal shedding or accumulation of stratum corneum is called scaling.

ULCER

An ulcer is a discontinuity of the epidermis affecting the pappillary dermis leading to scar formation.

VESICLE

It is a well-circumscribed elevated lesion that contains fiuid. It is less than 5 mm in diameter.

STRUCTURE OF THE SKIN

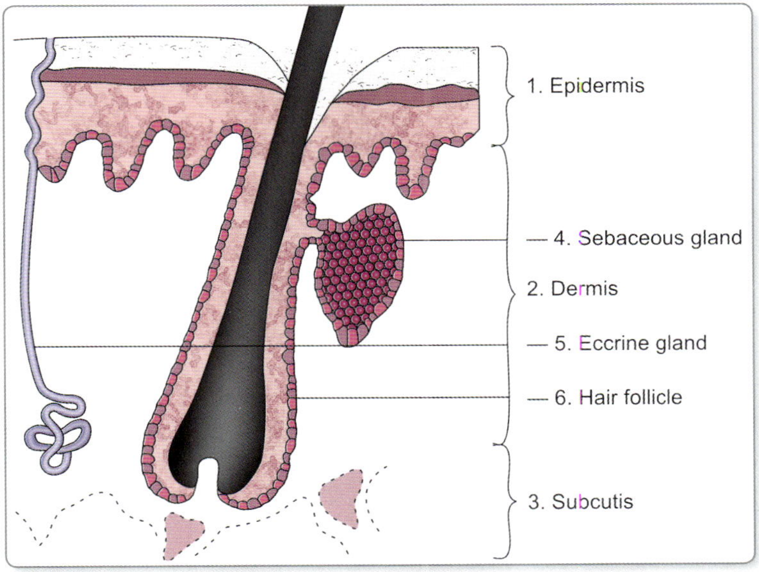

Structure of skin

Skin is divided into three layers; 1. Epidermis, 2. Dermis and 3. Subcutaneous tissue.

1. Epidermis

No blood vessels or lymphatics. Ectodermal origin. Basal cell layer, prickle cell layer, granular layer, clear cell layer, horny layer. Two types of cells: Keratinocytes, dendritic cells which include melanocytes. Langherhans' cells, indeterminate cells.

2. Dermis

Mesodermal origin, papillary dermis and reticular dermis, blood vessels, nerves, hairs and sweat and sebaceous glands present. Collagen fibers, reticulum fibers, elastic fibres and cells like mast cells, fibroblasts and histiocytes.

3. Subcutaneous Tissue

Mesodermal origin. Predominant cell is lipocyte, contains nerves, vessels, lymphatics, hair bulbs, coiled bodies of sweat glands; act as a heat regulator cushion against trauma, storage of nutritional energy.

FUNCTIONS OF THE SKIN

- Protective function, physical and chemical barrier.
- Thermoregulation
- Percutaneous absorption
- Sensory function
- Vitamin D synthesis.